AF696321

The Theory of Feverish Diseases and Its Clinical Applications

by
Hong-Yen Hsu
Su-Yen Wang

ORIENTAL HEALING ARTS INSTITUTE
1945 PALO VERDE AVE. SUITE 208
LONG BEACH, CA. 90815 U.S.A.

The Theory of Feverish Diseases and Its Clinical Applications

English Copyright 1985 by the Oriental Healing Arts Institute of the United States. No part of this book may be reproduced by any mechanical, photographic, or electronic process, or in the form of a photographic recording, nor may it be stored in a retrieval system, transmitted, or otherwise copied for public or private use – other than for "fair use" – without the written permission of the publisher.

ISBN: 0-941942-20-1
Printed in Taiwan, R.O.C.

Table of Contents

Notice

The following is a summary description of some of the natural herbal formulas widely used throughout Asia. The information compiled from traditional medical texts and from the observations of modern authorities on Chinese medicine is presented here for its educational value and should not be used for diagnosis, treatment, or prevention of disease without the advice of a Chinese physician or other medical authority.

Chinese version of this publication is available by mail from. . . . .

ORIENTAL HEALING ARTS INSTITUTE
1945 PALO VERDE AVE. SUITE 208
LONG BEACH, CA. 90815 U.S.A.

Foreword

In China and Southeast Asia the most important classics for the study of Chinese medicine are the *Nei ching* (The Yellow Emperor's Classic of Internal Medicine), the *Shang han lun* (Treatise on Febrile Diseases), the *Chin kuei yao lueh* (Prescriptions from the Golden Chamber), and the *Wen ping hsueh* (The Theory of Feverish Diseases). Of these the *Nei ching* has been partially translated into English and is readily available and the *Shang han lun* and *Chin kuei yao lueh* have been published by the Oriental Healing Arts Institute of U.S.A. The *Wen ping hsueh,* however, remains untranslated.

The *Shang han lun* theory speaks of the feverish diseases. To quote, "The condition of warm fever without chillphobia in the greater yang disease indicates a feverish disease." Since then, however, theories of feverish disease gradually evolved, developing into an independent discipline during the Ming and Ching dynasties and later splitting off and forming the *wen ping* school separate from the *shang han* school. Through generations, publications of *wen ping* have been growing in numbers and many of its duplications, commentaries, and translations have been widely circulated in Southeast Asia, China, Taiwan, and Japan. For the sake of clarification we will summarize some of the original works.

1. *Hsin kan wen ping* (新感温病 , Newly Contracted Feverish Diseases) by Wang Chi (汪機) of the Ming dynasty

Before publishing this famous book, Wang Chi (1493-1539

A.D.) had treated feverish diseases according to the theory presented by the *Nei ching:* "People afflicted by chills in the winter will develop fever the next spring." After thorough study, Wang found that feverish diseases occur immediately after one has been affected by external pathogenic factors and that *shang han* diseases – spring feverish disease, summer sunstroke, winter common cold, and dampness in the autumn – are not confined to a specific season. He then broke away from the *Shang han lun* theory by redefining another medical theory of feverish diseases.

2. *Wen yi hsueh* (温疫學, Theory of Plague) by Wu You-ko (吳又可) of the Ming dynasty

Wu You-ko (1592-1672 A.D.), also called Wu You-hsing, was an outstanding specialist in epidemic febrile diseases of the Ming dynasty. He carefully observed the characteristics and natures of various epidemic febrile diseases prevailing in 1641 and set forth his experience in the *Theory of Plague* in about 50,000 words. The book discussed pathology, etiology, epidemiology, and clinical findings of contagious diseases. He pointed out that febrile diseases and sunstroke are caused by the normal *ch'i* of nature, whereas plague results from *li ch'i* (厲氣, epidemic noxious factors). He further separated febrile diseases and epidemic febrile diseases into infectious and noninfectious diseases and concluded that all openings on the surface of the human body such as the mouth, nose, and skin provide an entrance for communicable pathogens which are carried to the openings by *li ch'i.*

3. *Wen je lun* (温熱論, Treatise on Feverish Diseases) by Yeh Tien-shih (葉天士) of the Ching dynasty

Yeh Tien-shih (1667-1746 A.D.), also known as Yeh Hsiang-yen, pointed out in this book that the pathogenic factors of an epidemic fever normally invade the lungs first and then adversely attack the pericardium, causing impairment of consciousness or coma. He spotted the medium of feverish diseases and summarized their relationship to protective *ch'i,* nutrients, and blood. He also listed therapeutic methods for wind dampness and feverish diseases. His insights opened the door for better treatment of acute diseases.

4. ***Wen ping tiao pien*** **(温病條辨 , Detailed Analysis of Feverish Diseases) by Wu Tang (吳瑭) of the Ching dynasty**

Wu Tang (1736-1829 A.D.), also known as Wu Chu-tung, had witnessed several kinds of epidemic diseases in his life. He set forth his experience in this book based on Yeh Tien-shih's *Treatise on Feverish Diseases.* In his book he concentrated on differential diagnosis of diseases according to pathological changes of the triple warmers, drew distinctions among spring, wind, summer, dampness, winter, and autumn feverish diseases, and listed methods of treatment. He systematized the *wen ping* theory.

5. ***Wen je ping pien*** **(温熱病篇 , Papers on Feverish Diseases) by Hsueh Sheng-pai (薛生白) of the Ching dynasty**

Hsueh Sheng-pai (1681-1770 A.D.), originally named Hsueh Hsueh, wrote these papers which, although lost, partially survived in other classics such as Wang Mong-ying's *The Longitude and Latitude of Feverish Diseases* (*Wen je ching wei* 温熱經緯). These papers dealt with pathological changes of dampness feverish diseases, differentiation of conformations, and methods of treatment in great detail. His observations greatly aided the study of this discipline in the subsequent generations. These papers and the *Detailed Analysis of Feverish Diseases* remain required classics for herbal practitioners.

6. ***Shih ping lun*** **(時病論 , On Seasonal Diseases) by Lei Feng (雷豐)**

Lei Feng (birth and death dates unknown), also called Lei Shao-yi, published this book in eight volumes in 1882. With this work he restructured feverish diseases described in *Su wen* (素問 , Simple Questions) into the pathologies of spring feverish disease, wind feverish disease, winter feverish disease, *shang han* disease, damp feverish disease, sunstroke, toxic feverish disease, autumn feverish disease, cough, diarrhea, and dysentery. He also stated the causes, symptoms, and treatment of the diseases and introduced his own prescriptions in addition to commonly employed older formulas.

7. ***Wen je ching wei* (温熱經緯 , The Longitude and Latitude of Feverish Diseases) by Wang Shih-hsiung (王士雄) of the Ching dynasty**

Wang Shih-hsiung (1809-1890 A.D.), also called Wang Mong-ying, wrote his book to explain the causes of feverish diseases, their signs and symptoms, and methods of treatment on the basis of the theories stated in the *Nei ching, Shang han lun,* and *Chin kuei yao lueh,* in comparison with the viewpoints of the distinguished physicians previously mentioned. He defined terms such as *wai kan* (外感 , external affection), *hsin kan* (新感 , new affection), and *fu ch'i* (伏氣, the latent pathogen), among others, to promote a better understanding of diseases and their treatment.

While many other authors wrote on feverish diseases, the above represent the main sources forming the basis of modern Chinese theory.

Wen ping comprises a category of external pathological diseases, a collective term for various acute febrile diseases caused by different warm pathogenic factors occurring in various seasons. According to this theory pathological changes are characterized by a relatively acute onset with heat signs predominant at the early stages that tend to damage bodily fluids and liquid essence. In some works, the infectious *wen ping* is termed *wen yi* (温疫 , plague) and noninfectious *wen ping* merely *wen ping.* This distinction may not be suitable for the conditions they bring about, but it does cast the term *wen ping* in a broader sense. Hence, *wen ping* (plague), in a narrow sense, should refer to highly contagious epidemic febrile diseases.

The theory of *wen ping* was barely introduced to Japan, owing to Japan's geographical location in the temperate and frigid zones where diseases were treated traditionally with prescriptions from the *Shang han lun* and *Chin kuei yao lueh,* Furthermore, the Ming and Ching periods in China coincided with the Tokugawa period of isolationism in Japan which greatly curtailed communication with the outside world, thus preventing this discipline from entering Japan. Nevertheless, the theory of *wen ping* is gaining acceptance in Japan today and some of the works have already been translated into Japanese.

We first planned to translate the *Theory of Feverish Diseases* into English, but considering that many of our readers are not familiar with this discipline, we decided to publish the book with particular emphasis on clinical applications. By compiling and editing the materials listed in the bibliography and drawing clinical applications from my previous book *An Outline of Differential Diagnosis* (Chinese) we created a suitable text for our purposes.

Representing a general concept of *wen ping* and its clinical applications, this book serves well for beginning practitioners interested in studying feverish diseases. Following this same goal we will publish the *Wen ping tiao pien* (温病條辨, Detailed Analysis of Feverish Diseases) and *Wen ping hsueh* (温病學, The Theory of Feverish Diseases) to enhance our readers' understanding. Modern physicians employ antimicrobial drugs on a very large scale in the treatment of feverish diseases. While their use brings striking therapeutic results, they can create serious complications, endanger the human body, and, in some cases, lead to death. We all know only too well that frequent and excessive use of these "magic bullets" renders bacterial strains resistant to antibiotics. Unfortunately herbal drugs which have been used for thousands of years in treating the same diseases, particularly those in the lesser yang stage, have not yet received their due. We hope concerned physicians will further study this discipline with a desire to integrate it with modern medicine. Should this book prove of heuristic value in joining Western science and Eastern wisdom, it has attained its goal.

I am indebted to Mr. Wang Su-yen for his translation and to Paul Laurence, associate editor, and Jeannine E. Talley, Ph.D., senior editor, for polishing the prose.

Los Angeles

Hong-yen Hsu
President, Oriental Healing Arts Institute
January 25, 1985

1
Introduction

In traditional Chinese medicine the term *wen ping* refers collectively to various feverish diseases including *tsun wen* (春温 spring feverish disease), *feng wen* (風温 wind feverish disease), *shu wen* (暑溫 summer feverish disease), *shih wen* (濕溫 moisture feverish disease), *fu shu* (伏暑 hidden summer feverish disease), *chiu tsao* (秋燥 autumn aridity feverish disease), *tung wen* (冬温 winter feverish disease), and *wen tu* (温毒 feverish toxin disease). These diseases differ in the seasons of occurrence, etiologies, and symptoms, but all have the same mechanism of pathological transmission. In ancient times, though very careful and detailed observations of the clinical symptoms had been made and the corresponding treatment methods developed, the disease itself was not described by means of pathological and physiological analyses and studies.

The term *wen ping* first appeared in the *Nei ching* (内經 The Yellow Emperor's Classic of Internal Medicine), later the *Nan ching* (難經 The Classic of Medical Difficulties), and the *Shang han lun* (傷寒論 A Treatise on Febrile Diseases). It is now briefly described as follows.

The *Nei ching* says, "One person afflicted by chills in the winter will develop fever the next spring," and "Affliction by chills that develops fever before the summer solstice is a feverish disease; chills after the summer solstice is a summer heat disease."

The *Nan ching* says, "There are five types of *shang han* diseases, namely: *chung feng* (中風 wind stroke), *shang han* (傷寒 chill injuries), *shih wen* (濕溫 moisture fever), *je ping* (熱病 fever disease), and *wen ping* (温病 feverish disease)." The greater yang chapter in the *Shang han lun* says, "The condition of fever with thirst but without chillphobia signals a feverish disease. The condition of generalized scorching fever after perspiration indicates a wind fever." These signs, however, only describe the diseases and do not suggest therapeutic methods. Wang Su-ho (王叔和) of the Tsin (晋) dynasty says in his *Shang han hsu* (傷寒序), "In the severe chill of the winter days, a contraction of chill that immediately develops into a disease is a *shang han* disease. If the chill does not cause a disease, it is hidden within the skin and muscles where it develops into a feverish disease the following spring. If the disease occurs in the summer, it is a summer fever, which has a higher fever than a feverish disease." Hence, subsequent people believed that feverish diseases derive from hidden chills. The *Chien chin fang* (千金方), written in the Tang dynasty, differentiates feverish diseases into *yang tu* (陽毒 yang toxin) and *yin tu* (陰毒 yin toxin) types, depending on whether they afflict the luminal (腑 *fu*) or solid (臟 *tsang*) viscera, and says wind feverish disease can be treated with *Wei-jui-tang* (葳蕤湯 Polygonatum and Mahuang Combination). This is the first recorded treatment for feverish diseases. The *Shang han tsung ping lun* (傷寒總論病) by Pang An-shih (龐安時) of the Sung dynasty and the *Lei cheng huo jen shu* (類證活人書) by Chu Kung (朱肱) both clearly point out that the feverish diseases differ from the *shang han* diseases in their methods of treatment. Liu Ho-chien (劉河間) of the Chin (金) and Yuan (元) dynasties contends that all the diseases altered from the *shang han* diseases via the six meridians are fever diseases. He invented *Shuang-chieh-san* (雙解散 Siler and Mentha Formula) and *Liang-ke-san* (涼膈散 Forsythia and Rhubarb Formula), among others, formulas that resolve both the surface and the interior. Subsequent people regard him as the initiator of treatment of feverish diseases. However, his theory is still not free from the bondage of the *Shang han lun*. In the Ming (明) dynasty, Wu You-ko (吳又可), in his *Wen i lun* (温疫論 Exposition on Feverish Plagues) had already realized that feverish diseases are contagious. By the time of the Ching (清) dynasty the feverish disease theories had coalesced into an independent theoretical system comprised of two major schools—the *shang han* and feverish disease schools, as represented by the following examples.

1. Yeh Tien-shih (葉天士) wrote *Wen je lun* (温熱論 Treatise on Feverish Diseases) in which he proposed the theory of *wei* (衛 protective), *ch'i* (氣 *ch'i*), *ying* (營 viscerovascular), and *hsueh* (血 blood) systems, by which he identified conformations and argued about methods of treatment. He thus developed the diagnostic methods for feverish diseases.

2. Wu Chu-tung (吳鞠通), in his *Wen ping tiao pien* (温病條辨 upon which we have based this English version) added his own supplements to Yeh's theoretical foundation.

3. Wang Mong-ying (王孟英) wrote *Wen ping ching wei* (温病經緯 The Longitude and Latitude of Feverish Diseases) by referring to the *Nei ching* and the *Shang han lun* and summarizing Yeh Tien-shih's theory.

The distinctive differences in conformation and treatment between the *shang han* and feverish diseases are shown in Table 1.

Additional clinical observations are summarized in Table 2.

2
Conformations in Terms of *Wei*, *Ch'i*, *Ying*, and *Hsueh*

To identify the conformations of feverish diseases one must grasp the developmental processes of the diseases. In this area Yeh Tien-shih of the Chin dynasty was influenced by Liu Wan-su's and Wu You-ko's theories. He wrote *Wen je lun* (Treatise on Feverish Diseases) in which he divided the development of feverish diseases into four stages–*wei* (衛), *ch'i* (氣), *ying* (營) and *hsueh* (血)–and said:

> Generally speaking, *ch'i* comes after *wei*, and *hsueh* after *ying*. When a feverish disease is in the *wei* stage, it can be treated by the sweating method. Only when it is in the *ch'i* stage can the *ch'i* be cleaned. When it enters the ying stage, we can treat it by driving out the fever and transferring the *ch'i*. If the disease has entered the blood stage however, this kind of treatment will waste and violate the blood. The treatment then

Table 1. Comparison of *Shang han* and Feverish Diseases at the Initial Stage; Conformation and Treatment

<table>
<tr><th colspan="3">Disease type</th><th>Shang han</th><th>Feverish</th></tr>
<tr><td colspan="3">Etiology</td><td>Chills penetrate body surface to cause suppression and confinement of protective yang</td><td>Fever contracted in upper torso, hinders normal functioning of protective ch'i</td></tr>
<tr><td rowspan="8">Conformation</td><td colspan="2">Fever</td><td>Relatively mild</td><td>Relatively severe</td></tr>
<tr><td colspan="2">Chillphobia</td><td>Severe</td><td>Mild</td></tr>
<tr><td colspan="2">Headache, body ache</td><td>Severe</td><td>Mild</td></tr>
<tr><td colspan="2">Thirst</td><td>No</td><td>Slight</td></tr>
<tr><td colspan="2">Urine</td><td>Clear, profuse</td><td>Yellowish</td></tr>
<tr><td rowspan="2">Tongue</td><td>Color</td><td>Normal</td><td>Red on apex and ridge</td></tr>
<tr><td>Fur</td><td>White</td><td>White</td></tr>
<tr><td colspan="2">Pulse</td><td>Floating, tense</td><td>Floating, quick</td></tr>
<tr><td colspan="3">Treatment rule</td><td>Use acrid and warm herbs to produce sweating</td><td>Use acrid and cool herbs to resolve surface</td></tr>
</table>

Table 2. Comparison of *Shang han* and Feverish Diseases; General Characteristics

Shang han	Feverish
Occurs promptly upon contracting.	Occurs after contracting with indefinite latency period.
Chill evils enter through hair and pores.	Feverish evils enter via mouth and nose.
Chill evils enter interior from surface.	Feverish evils go from superior to inferior.
Chill evils conceive normal *ch'i* of world.	Feverish evils conceive severe, pathological *ch'i* of world.
Do not infect other people.	Infect other people.
Chillphobia present from onset.	No chillphobia or mild chillphobia in beginning.
No interior fever in beginning when disease is on surface.	Interior fever from very beginning.
Pulse is floating and tense, or floating and moderate.	Pulse is floating and quick, or surging and quick.
Yang is liable to get injured.	Yin is liable to get injured.
Treated with acrid and warm herbs to induce perspiration.	Treat with acrid and cool herbs to resolve muscles.
Only treat surface with sweating method, but avoid violating interior.	Treat surface with sweating method, and frequently also purge interior.
Sweating treatment is never too early.	Sweating treatment is never too late.
Purgation is never too late.	Purgation is never too early.
Purge dry, hard stool.	Purge suppressed fever.
Purgation conducted only when all surface symptoms have disappeared.	Purgation is conducted in simultaneous presence of surface and internal conformations.
One purgation is always enough.	Frequently repeated purgation is required.

is to cool and disperse the blood.

Generally, when a feverish disease at its onset exhibits fever and slight chillphobia, it is in the *wei* stage. If it exhibits fever, absence of chillphobia, and yellow urine, it is in the *ch'i* stage. If it exhibits a quick pulse and a red tongue, it has entered the *ying* stage. If the tongue is dark red and the patient is irritable, unable to sleep or has delirium at night, the disease has advanced into the blood stage.

The principal symptoms of the four stages follows:

The *wei* stage conformation is frequently observed at the beginning of a feverish disease. The clinical manifestations are fever, slight anemophobia and chillphobia, headache, anhidrosis or oligohidrosis, cough, thirst, thin tongue fur, red apex and ridge of the tongue, and a floating and quick pulse. Of these symptoms, fever, slight anemophobia and chillphobia, anhidrosis, and a floating and quick pulse comprise the basic characteristics of this stage. Because the lungs are associated with the skin and hair and the *wei* (protective or skin) system communicates with the lung *ch'i,* when the lungs and the *wei* system are in disharmony, cough and thirst also occur.

The *ch'i* stage conformation includes a wide range of symptoms with fever, absence of chillphobia, thirst, and yellow tongue fur being the basic ones. As illness evils enter the *ch'i* stage, they antagonize the normal *ch'i;* the fever so generated suppresses the function of the *ch'i,* causing disordered *ch'i* functioning and injuries in the related viscera.

If the illness evils are not resolved in the *ch'i* stage, they will advance into the *ying* stage; or if the patient's normal *ch'i* is empty and weakened and his bodily fluids become depleted, evils from the *ch'i* stage will go adversely into the *ying* (viscerovascular system) stage where the fever generated will cause a dark red tongue, annoyance in the heart, insomnia, frequent delirium, a generalized fever growing severe at night, no serious thirst, macules slightly visible beneath the skin, and a thin, quick pulse. Among these symptoms the most characteristic are generalized fever growing severe at night, a dark red tongue, annoyance in the heart, and delirium. The pathological changes caused by evils in the *ying* stage are expressed in two ways—fever injuring *ying's* yin (visceral substantials) and a disturbed heart and spirit.

The *hsueh* stage conformation results when the illness evils in the *ying* stage remain unresolved and progress farther toward the blood stage. As the fever enters the blood, it manifests a generalized fever, causing irritability and annoyance, or even madness and craziness, a dark red tongue, hematemesis, epistaxis, hematuria, bloody stool, accumulated blood, and densely spread macules. Among these symptoms, a dark red tongue and bleeding are most characteristic. Since the heart controls the blood and stores the spirit, when feverish evil invades the blood, it manifests a thriving fever disturbing the blood and offending the heart and spirit.

The conformational manifestations of *wei, ch'i, ying,* and *hsueh* reflect the depth of the feverish evil location and the severity of the disease as indicated in Table 3. The *wei* stage is the most shallow location of the evil and the mildest disease. The *ch'i* stage indicates the disease has advanced into the interior. The pathological changes in the *ch'i* stage occur in the lungs, chest, diaphragm, stomach, intestines, gallbladder and spleen. These diseases prove more severe than those of the *wei* stage. At this stage the normal *ch'i* remains exuberant and strongly resistant to evils. Even though the disease is fierce, the evil can be easily driven out and the disease cured if treatment begins in time. As the fever evil moves further into the *ying* and *hsueh* stages, it not only wastes and injures viscerovascular blood but also affects the spirit. The disease in these stages is the severest.

3
Conformations of the Three Warmers

Being influenced by the theories of Yeh Tien-shih and others, Wu Tang (Chu-tung) proposed in his *Wen ping tiao pien* (温病條辨) that *shang han* diseases derive from water and feverish disease from fire. On the basis of this theory, he established the rule of treating feverish diseases: cleanse the fever and nourish

Table 3. Comparison of *Wei, Ch'i, Ying,* and *Hsueh* Disease Stages; *Chi* Contingencies: No Chillphobia Versus Thermophobia

Disease Stage	Symptoms		Treatment rule	Indicated formulas
	Characteristic	Other		
Wei	Fever, chillphobia	Head, body ache, cough, pharyngeal ache, floating-quick pulse, white tongue fur	Use acrid, cool herbs to resolve surface	*Sang-chu-yin-chia-chien* (桑菊飲加減 Morus and Chrysanthemum Combination modified)
Ch'i	Fever, no chillphobia, yet thermophobia	Sweating, thirst, puffing, surging, big and quick pulse, yellow tongue fur	Clean *ch'i* and detoxify	*Pai-hu-tang* (白虎湯 Gypsum Combination) combined with *Sang-chu-yin* (桑菊飲)
		Tidal fever, ruddy face, abdominal distention, discomfort upon abdominal pressing, constipation, diarrhea, anal burning, submerged and forceful pulse	Purge and dispel toxin	*Ta-cheng-chi-tang* (大承氣湯 Major Rhubarb Combination)
Ying	Dark red tongue	Dark red tongue without fur, no thirst, unconsciousness, delirium, stiff tongue, convulsions, thin, quick pulse	Cleanse *ying*, purge fever, clean heart, open up cavities	*Tou-je-chuan-chi-tang* (透熱轉氣湯 Gypsum and Anemone Combination)
Hsueh	Purplish red tongue	Eruption of macules, bleeding tendency	Cool and arrest blood	*Liang-hsueh-pai-tu-tang* (涼血敗毒湯 Lonicera and Gypsum Combination)

the yin. He attributed the etiologies to the three warmers, with each warmer governing certain viscera.

The symptoms of feverish diseases as manifested in the three warmers are:

Upper warmer symptoms: Symptoms of this warmer are essentially the pathological changes of the hand-greater yin-lung meridian and the hand-absolute yin-pericardium meridian. When the condition is due to ill evils present in the hand-greater yin-lungs meridian, the *wei ch'i* is suppressed and the functions of the lungs and *wei* system are hindered. The resulting symptoms include fever, chillphobia, anhidrosis or oligohidrosis, slight thirst, cough, floating and quick pulse, thin and white tongue fur, and redness at the ridge and apex of the tongue. If surface evils enter into the interior and result in the lungs becoming congested with evil fever and hinder the functioning of the lung *ch'i,* the symptoms manifested are generalized fever, perspiration, thirst, cough, asthma, yellow tongue fur, and a quick pulse. If it is due to a feverish evil entering the hand-absolute yin-pericardium meridian, causing a blocking of functional cavities, the symptoms are unconsciousness, delirium, loss of sensation with aphrasia, stiff tongue, limbic chills, and a dark red tongue.

Middle warmer symptoms: These symptoms represent the pathological changes of the foot-sunlight yang-stomach, hand-sunlight yang-colon, and foot-greater yin-spleen meridians. The stomach, a yang organ, and the spleen, a yin organ, are located in the middle warmer region of the body (torso). The former controls aridity and the latter, moisture. If the evil that enters the middle warmer is converted by and into aridity, the symptoms are fever without chillphobia but with thermophobia; aggravation of this condition at dusk; hyperemia in the face and eyes; a low, unclear voice; labored breathing; constipation; pain when urinating; and yellow or even parched black tongue fur with spikes, indicating the presence of a firm fever. If the evil entering the middle warmer is converted by and into moisture, the symptoms are mild but stable somatic fever, distention and distress in the chest and stomach, nausea, generalized heaviness and limbic fatigue, greasy tongue fur, and a moderate pulse, all of which indicate a moisture feverish conformation.

Lower warmer symptoms: These symptoms derive chiefly from the pathological changes of the foot-lesser yin-kidney meridian and the foot-absolute yin-liver meridian. The symptoms include lingering stomachic fever, and, in case the genuine yin of the kidneys (visceral substantials) is injured, generalized fever, facial hyperemia, higher fever on the palms and soles than on the back sides of the hands and feet, dry mouth and throat, an empty pulse, fatigued spirit, and vexation in the heart causing insomnia. If the renal yin is exhausted, the hepatic wood is not nourished and becomes weakened. The weakened wood then develops an internally moving wind that causes the symptoms of limbic vermication or even spasms and flaccidity, a fatigued spirit, limbic chilling, cardiac palpitation, a dark red tongue with little fur, and an empty and weak pulse. Feverish evils readily injure the yin (visceral substantials) and exhaust humors. Hence, when a feverish disease is transmitted to the lower warmer, the symptoms are mostly due to yin weakness of the liver and the kidneys.

Generally the transmission and variation of the visceral conformations of the three warmers begins in the hand-greater yin-lung meridian of the upper warmer. If the conformation is transmitted to the middle warmer, it is a normal transmission. If it is transmitted to the pericardium, it is an adverse transmission. The occurrence of adverse transmission is determined by both the evils and the normal *ch'i.* Generally, deficient cardiac *ch'i* or deficient cardiac yin and contraction of severe evils cause adverse transmission. When the disease is not healed at the middle warmer it is transmitted to the liver and kidneys of the lower warmer. This is the condition of common transmission, but it is not fixed and unchangeable. In the process of transmission, in some cases the middle warmer conformation appears while the upper warmer remains unresolved, and in other cases the lower warmer conformation may appear before the middle warmer conformation is eliminated.

The conformations of diseases of the three warmers are summarized in Table 4.

Table 4. Conformations and Treatments of Diseases of the Three Warmers

Warmer	Meridian	Main symptoms	Treatment rule	Indicated formulas
Upper	Hand-greater yin-lungs	Fever, chillphobia, cough, headache	Acrid, cool herbs to resolve surface	*Sang-chu-yin* (桑菊飲 Morus and Chrysanthemum Combination)
	Hand-absolute yin-pericardium	Unconsciousness, delirium, red tongue, convulsions, fainting, spasms, flaccidity	Cleanse heart and open up cavities	*Tung-chiao-hsi-feng-tang* (通竅熄風湯 Haliotis and Gentiana Combination)
Middle	Foot-sunlight yang-stomach	Fever without chillphobia, sweating, thirst, quick-big pulse	Cleanse fever and save body fluids	*Chu-yeh-shih-kao-tang* (竹葉石膏湯 Bamboo Leaf and Gypsum Combination)
	Foot-greater yin-spleen	Low stable somatic fever, thoracic depression, nausea, bodily distress, moderate pulse, greasy tongue fur	Cleanse fever and resolve turbidity	*San-jen-tang-chia-chien* (三仁湯加減 Apricot, Coix, and Cluster Combination modified) *Huo-pu-hsia-ling-tang* (藿朴夏苓湯 Agastache and Polyporus Combination)
Lower	Foot-lesser yin-kidney	Somatic fever, facial hyperemia, higher fever on palms and soles than on back sides of hands and feet, vexation in heart causing insomnia	Nourish blood and yin	*Ching-ying-tang* (清營湯 Rhinoceros and Scrophularia Combination)
	Foot-absolute yin-liver	Cardiac palpitation, limbic vermication, even spasms and flaccidity	Nourish the liver and quiet wind	*Ah-chiao-chih-tzu-huang-tang* (阿膠雞子黃湯 Gelatin and Yolk Combination) *Ta-ting-feng-chu* (大定風珠 Peony and Gelatin Formula)

4
Differences and Similarities of *Wei, Ch'i, Ying, Hsueh,* and *San Chiao* Conformations

The conformational identifications in terms of *wei, ch'i, ying, hsueh,* and *san chiao* or in terms of the six meridians are basically similar. Both identification methods are used for explaining the severity and depth of illness evils. While the *san chiao* method divides the locations of the illness evils into three areas and holds that the feverish disease evil enters our bodies through the mouth or nose and is transmitted from the superior to the inferior part of the body, the six meridians method describes the evils entering the body from the surface to the interior or going from shallow to deep. Both theories are alike in that one views the evils vertically from the upper to the lower part, and the other horizontally from the outside to the inside. However, there are differences between the two. For example, the pathological change of the upper warmer's hand-greater yin-lung meridian is equivalent to a condition of evils located in the *wei* stage. If fever is trapped in the lungs without a manifestation of surface conformation, the condition belongs to the *ch'i* stage. While the pathological change resulting from fever entering the pericardium can be included in the *ying* stage, the symptomatic manifestations vary. In the initial period of this stage, the condition is phlegmic fever obstructed internally; in the later period it is fever injuring the visceral substantials. Also, the pathological changes of the middle warmer's foot-sunlight yang-stomach meridian and foot-greater yin-spleen meridian are within the *ch'i* stage, though the condition of evils remaining in the *ch'i* stage is not restricted to pathological changes of the middle warmer. Any condition with evils existing neither on the surface nor in the interior can be included in the *ch'i* stage. The pathological changes and evils of the liver and kidneys in the lower warmer are in the blood stage. However, the conformations exhibited are differentiated into firm and weak. From the above, we see that in clinical application both methods of conformational identification should be combined so that we can use them to direct our identification of conformations, and prescribe the proper treatment. The theory of feverish diseases and the theory of *shang han* diseases are compared in Table 5.

Table 6 compares the conformations and main pathological changes of feverish diseases using the eight principles and the four disease stages methods.

5
Relationships Between Feverish Diseases and the Weather of the Four Seasons

Due to seasonal weather changes and differences in individual personal constitutions, feverish diseases also differ in clinical symptomatic manifestations and course of development. Therefore, Chinese physicians delving into the research of feverish diseases divide the diseases into various types in accordance with the different seasonal climates. The symptoms and characteristics of these feverish diseases are as follows.

A. Wind feverish disease: This type of feverish disease occurs mostly in the spring and the winter (that occurring in the winter is also called winter feverish disease). At the onset, the symptoms are chiefly fever, slight anemophobia, chillphobia, cough, and thirst. Generally the external wind and fever evils are contracted and enter the body via the mouth and nose. After entering the body, the evils first offend the lungs. Since the lungs are in charge of the *ch'i* belonging to the *wei* domain and associated with the skin and hair system, the beginning symptoms are those of the lungs and *wei* domain. The disease advances toward the stomach and intestine (which is normal transmission) or toward the pericardium (which is adverse transmission).

B. Spring feverish disease: This type of feverish disease occurs in the spring. An internal fever conformation appears right from the beginning. The etiologies of this disease are differentiated

Table 5. Comparison of *Shang han,* Wind-feverish, Summer-feverish and Moisture-feverish Diseases

Disease type	Onset season	Symptoms	Treatment rule	Indicated formulas
Shang han	Winter	Initially there is more chillphobia than fever, headache, body ache, anhidrosis, floating-tense or floating-moderate pulse, thin white tongue fur	Use acrid warm herbs to produce sweating	*Ma-huang-tang* (麻黄湯 Mahuang Combination) *Kuei-chih-tang* (桂枝湯 Cinnamon Combination)
		When evil has been transmitted to interior there is fever without chillphobia, fast-big pulse, yellow tongue fur	Cleanse surface of sunlight-yang meridian	*Pai-hu-tang* (白虎湯 Gypsum Combination)
		Tidal fever, annoying thirst, distention in stomach and abdomen, submerged-full pulse, thick yellow or thick dark red tongue fur	Purge	*Ta-cheng-ch'i-tang* (大承氣湯 Major Rhubarb Combination)
		Alternating chills and fever, chordal-slippery pulse	Harmonize	*Hsiao-chai-hu-tang* (小柴胡湯 Minor Bupleurum Combination)
		Fever without chillphobia or slight chillphobia in beginning, thirst, cough, pharyngeal ache, hidrosis or anhidrosis, mild headache, vomiting, red tongue, thin white tongue fur	Use acrid cool herbs to resolve surface	*Sang-chu-yin* (桑菊飲 Morus and Chrysanthemum Combination) *Yin-chiao-san* (銀翹散 Lonicera and Forsythia Formula)

Table 5. Continued

Disease type	Onset season	Symptoms	Treatment rule	Indicated formulas
Wind-feverish	Any season, especially spring	Fever without chillphobia, thirst, vexation and irritability, spontaneous perspiration, ruddy face, puffing breaths, slippery pulse, red tongue, yellow or dark red tongue fur	Cleanse fever and detoxify poisons	*Tseng-shun-san-huang-shih-kao-tang* (增損三黃石膏湯 Gypsum, Coptis, and Scute Combination modified)
		Unconsciousness and delirium	Use fragrant herbs to open cavities	*An-kung-niu-huang-wan* (安宮牛黃丸 Bos and Curcuma Formula)
		Distention of stomach and abdomen, constipation	Resolve both surface and interior	*Tseng-shun-shuan-chieh-san* (增損雙解散 Siler and Mentha Formula modified)
Summer-feverish	Summer	Sudden onset of high fever, headache, vomiting, severe thirst, craving for water, hyperhidrosis, vexation, irritation and unease, comatose sleep, ruddy face, thin white tongue fur, slippery-quick or soft-quick pulse	Cleanse *ch'i* and relieve muscles	*Ching-shu-chieh-tu-tang* (清暑解毒湯 Lonicera and Anemarrhena Combination)
		If accompanied by unconsciousness, delirium, spasms and palsy, convulsions, dark-red tongue, yellow fur, surging quick pulse	Open cavities, extinguish winds	*Tung-chiao-hsi-feng-tang* (通竅熄風湯) Haliotis and Gentiana Combination)

Table 5. Continued

Disease type	Onset season	Symptoms	Treatment rule	Indicated formulas
		If there is tidal fever, hyperhidrosis, ruddy face and eyes, abdominal distention, constipation or dark brown muddy stool with stinking odor	Use purgation to dispel toxin	*Pai-hu-cheng-chi-tang* (Gypsum, Rhubarb, and Anemarrhena Combination 白虎承氣湯)
Moisture feverish	Between late summer and early autumn	Persisting fever becoming severer in the afternoon, pale yellow and greasy facial complexion, dull facial expression, thoracic depression without sensation of hunger, thirst without desire to drink or abdominal distention after drinking, heavy-headedness like the head being bound, lethargy, depressed, quick, inactive pulse, white greasy tongue fur	Use fragrant herbs to dissolve turbidity Use bitter, chilly herbs to cleanse fever	*San-jen-tang* (三仁湯 Apricot, Coix, and Cluster Combination) *Kan-lu-hsiao-tu-tan* (甘露消毒丹 Talc and Scute Formula)

Table 6. Summary of Stages, Conformations and Main Pathological Changes of Feverish Diseases

Feverish disease stage	Conformation identification method				Main symptoms	Tendency of changes	Main pathological changes
	Eight principles	Three warmers	*Wei, ch'i ying, hsueh*	Viscera			
Anemophobia	Surface, firm, fever	Upper warmer	*Wei*	Lungs	Chills, fever, cough	Mainly defensive reaction	Equivalent to symptoms of preliminary stage of acute contagious diseases and early stage when symptoms are eminent. Main changes are upper respiratory tract inflammation and peripheral neurovascular reactions
Fever development	Interior, firm, fever	Upper warmer, lower resistance	*Ch'i*	Lungs, stomach, intestine	Fever, constipation, injured fluids	Defensive reaction, pathological injuries begin to increase in severity	Equivalent to imminent symptom stage of acute contagious disease; humoral and electrolytic disturbances as the main change. Visceral parenchymatous turbidity, swelling, and functional disorders are present as specific pathological changes

Table 6. Continued

Feverish disease stage	Conformation identification method				Main symptoms	Tendency of changes	Main pathological changes
	Eight principles	Three warmers	*Wei, ch'i ying, hsueh*	Viscera			
Ying-intruding	Interior, firm, fever	Upper and middle warmer	*Ying*	Stomach, pericardium	Unconsciousness, macular eruption, bleeding	Defensive reaction begins to deteriorate, pathological injuries are main changes	Equivalent to culminant stage of acute contagious disease. In addition to further aggravation of specific changes of infectious diseases, CNS denaturization and necrosis become outstanding. Upsets blood coagulation process and further injures blood vessel walls due to poisoning
Yin-injury	Interior, weak, fever	Lower warmer	*Hsueh*	Liver, kidneys	Yin injury, spasmic faint	Decompensation begins until prostration	Equivalent to prostration stage of acute contagious diseases, more aggravated injuries in vital organs such as CNS, heart, lungs, kidneys, and liver. Organic reactivity and resistivity decline. Fulminative symptoms such as acute renal deficiency and diffusive bleeding are frequently exhibited

into "spontaneous occurrence of latent *ch'i*" and "occurrence induced by new contracting". If the feverish disease originates in the *ch'i* domain or *ch'i* stage, there will be *ch'i* fever injuring fluids or firm conformation with the sunlight yang viscera. If the disease originates in the *ying* domain or stage, the early symptoms are vexation, irritability, delirium, or even such a critical symptom as unconsciousness. This disease is due to a thriving internal fever which during the process of pathological changes is liable to cause agitation of winds and in the later stage often exhibits injured yin caused by the thriving fever, leading to maculation.

C. Summer feverish disease: This type of disease occurs in the summer, after the summer solstice. It is dramatic and exhibits right from the beginning the *ch'i* stage symptoms of strong fever, annoying thirst, and profuse sweating. Clinically, the illness is divided into summer fever and summer moisture diseases. The former, being of summer's fire-heat evil, is transmitted rapidly and exhibits from the beginning the symptoms of evils characteristic of the *ch'i* stage by skipping the *wei* stage. Hence, Yeh Tien-shih said, "The summer fever derives from the sunlight yang meridians." Summer fever most easily exhibits *ch'i* injury, humoral exhaustion, and even the critical symptom of humors and *ch'i* being at the verge of prostration. Because in the summer both temperature and moisture are very high, the disease exhibits not only summer fever but also generalized heaviness, distention of the stomach, and greasy tongue fur, which are obstructed moisture symptoms. Besides, in the summer people like to cool themselves with cool air or water or by drinking cold beverages, thereby suppressing summer moisture evils and exhibiting surface-chilling symptoms. Other diseases which resemble summer feverish diseases are:

1. Summer faint disease: The summer fever causes congestion of body cavities, causing sudden fainting and limbic chills.
2. Summer wind disease: Summer fever induces movement and agitation of internal wind, causing sudden fainting and convulsions.
3. Summer phthisis disease: Summer fever injures the lungs, resulting in an annoying fever, hemoptysis, or cough.

4. Summer filth disease: Filth obstructs clean cavities, resulting in the chief symptoms of vexation with depression, vomiting, nausea, or even fainting and unconsciousness.

D. Moisture feverish disease: This type of feverish disease is seen mostly in the period between the summer and the autumn, or during the plum-rain season (usually mid-summer with lingering rain for more than one month). It is transmitted relatively slowly and takes a longer period to develop. At the onset, external evils suppress the yang of the *wei* system, with *wei* stage symptoms such as chillphobia, heaviness and pain of the head and body, and also *ch'i*–stage symptoms resulting from suppressed and accumulated moisture evil such as stomachic distention and greasy tongue fur. As the surface conformation disappears, the disease will manifest as one of two distinct types: 1) more moisture than fever, and 2) more fever than moisture. The former condition exhibits lingering somatic fever, incessant sweating, thirst without desire to drink or with desire for hot drinks, chest depression causing nausea, bodily heaviness and limbic lassitude, watery stool, greasy white tongue fur, and a soft-moderate pulse. The latter condition exhibits generalized fever, bitter mouth, thirst without copious drinking, depressed stomach with retching, vexation in the heart, red urine, dark red color at the apex and ridges of the tongue, greasy yellow tongue fur, and a soft-quick pulse. Besides, moisture fever that is suppressed and steaming within the musculature and skin may cause leukoderma; that internally fumigating the liver and gallbladder may cause jaundice; that covering up the clear cavities of the upper body may cause insanity or unconsciousness; that stagnated in the urinary bladder in the lower body may lead to oliguria; that remaining unresolved may be transformed into an aridity evil which then accumulates in the sunlight yang area or injures the intestinal tract, leading to bloody stool.

E. Hidden summer heat feverish disease: This disease occurs in between the autumn and winter. Initially it resembles a common cold accompanied by summer heat and a moisture conformation. It then resembles malaria with irregular chills and fever.

Finally it exhibits a fever but no chills – the condition worsening at night but improving after perspiration in the day – incessant burning fever in the chest and abdomen, and diarrheal stool many times per day. Wu Chu-tung said, "Hidden summer heat, summer feverish, and moisture feverish diseases all derive from the same etiology. We must compare one to the others and avoid adhering rigidly to any one of them." In other words, the three conformations have the same pathological cause, hence in principle the treatment method for all three is the same. Generally, a condition with more summer fever than moisture can be treated according to the method for summer feverish disease, and a condition with more moisture than summer fever can be treated the same as for moisture-feverish diseases. In all, the three conditions can be compared to one another with respect to their conformations and treatment, but must nonetheless be clearly distinguished (see Table 7).

F. Autumn aridity feverish disease: This disease occurs in the autumn following a contraction of aridity evil. Although the disease is differentiated into cool aridity and feverish aridity types at the initial stage, it is caused by aridity evil in both types. Hence, in clinical manifestation, both types are very liable to show symptoms of dryness. As the disease condition changes and enters the sunlight yang stage, the patient develops intestinal aridity and constipation. If the disease goes further down into the lower warmer, it may cause injury to the yin *ch'i,* even though the evil fever is not strong. These manifestations appear the same as those of the other feverish diseases, yet their treatments are not exactly the same.

G. Feverish toxin: Contraction of feverish toxic vapor causes diseases with the characteristic symptoms of reddening, swelling, fever, and pain: for example, mumps, facial erysipelas, and diphtheria.

H. Feverish plague: A highly infectious disease, it is typically transmitted in epidemic fashion. Nevertheless, it exhibits the same symptoms. This disease is named feverish plague with an

Table 7. Comparison of Summer Feverish, Moisture Feverish and Hidden Summer Heat Diseases

Disease type	Onset season	Etiology	Mechanism	Conformation characteristics	Pulse	Tongue	Treatment rule
Summer feverish	Summer	Summer heat	Summer heat readily injures *ch'i*, hence symptoms are mostly internal fever, with injured *ch'i*.	Strong fever, polydipsia, profuse sweating, distention in head	Chordal, quick	Red with little fur	Cleanse *ch'i* fever, replenish yin *ch'i*
Moisture feverish	Long summer (between summer and autumn) and early autumn	Summer moisture	Moisture injures spleen and stomach in lingering condition	Generalized fever in afternoon like yin-weakness conformation, greasy mouth without thirst, constipation, short and harsh urination	Soft quick	Greasy, filthy with dark red color at apex and ridges	Resolve moisture and cleanse fever
Hidden summer heat	Very late autumn, winter	Summer moisture	Evils are located in mesentery or *ying* stage and converted into fever after long stagnation; lingering condition	Inconspicuous chills and fever like malaria, burning fever in chest and abdomen, constipation or diarrhea, short and harsh urination	Chordal, quick, languid	Greasy, filthy with dark red color at apex and ridges. Fur regrows after resolution	Cleanse internal fever and cause hidden evil to come out

intention to call people's attention to the severity of the disease and thus its prevention and treatment.

The above differentiation has theoretically divided feverish diseases into two classes: new contractions and hidden evils. The former refers to a new contraction of an external evil, which first exhibits a surface conformation such as fever, anemophobia or chillphobia, and then enters the interior from the surface, or goes from shallow to deep and undergoes gradual development. The latter, the hidden evil, does not manifest at the time of the contraction of the external evil. It begins inside the body and moves toward the outside after a latent period; characteristically it does not exhibit a prominent surface conformation at the onset. It begins right with the internal conformation, and emerges violently into a very severe disease condition. Spring feverish disease and hidden summer feverish disease belong to this class.

Classification by etiology divides feverish diseases into two categories–feverish fever and moisture fever diseases. The former category, like wind feverish, spring feverish, summer feverish, and autumn aridity diseases has a prompt onset, changes quickly, and tends to manifest a severe fever. Whereas the latter, like moisture feverish, hidden summer feverish, and feverish plague diseases results from the combination of fever and moisture evils, which then become stagnated in the *ch'i* domain for a longer time, thereby hindering the transforming function of the spleen and stomach.

6
Treatment of Feverish Diseases

According to the *Chung i pien cheng kan yao* (Outlines of Conformational Identification in Chinese Herbal Medicine) and *Wen ping hsueh chiang i* (Lectures on Feverish Diseases), treatment of the aforementioned feverish diseases can be effected on the basis of the *wei, ch'i, ying,* and *hsueh* classification principle as follows:

Table 8. Comparison of *Wei, Ch'i, Ying,* and *Hsueh* Stages of Wind-feverish Disease

Stage		Conformation			Treatment		
		Chief symptoms	Pulse	Tongue	Rule	Indicated formulas	Formula modification
Wei		Headache, somatic fever, chillphobia, slight thirst, cough	Floating, quick	White fur	Use acrid-cool herbs to resolve the surface	*Yin-chiao-san* (銀翹散 Lonicera and Forsythia Formula) *Sang-chu-yin* (桑菊飲 Morus and Chrysanthemum Combination)	For cough, add fritillaria, apricot seed, and eriobotrya; for yin weakness add raw fresh rehmannia
Ch'i	Evil fever obstructs the lungs	Cough, asthma, somatic fever, polydipsia	Quick	Red tongue, yellow fur	Disperse the lungs, cleanse fever	*Ma-hsing-kan-shih-tang* (麻杏甘石湯 Mahuang and Apricot Seed Combination) *Pai-hu-tang* (白虎湯)	
	Fever scorches sunlight yang	Strong fever, polydipsia	Surging, quick	Yellow fur	Use acrid-chilly herbs to cleanse *ch'i*	*Pai-hu-tang* (白虎湯 Gypsum Combination)	
	Fever accumulates in the stomach	Tidal fever, constipation, asthma and gasping with uneasiness	Forceful and big on right *chun*	Yellow fur	Disperse lungs and unblock luminal viscera	*Hsuan-pai-cheng-chi-tang** (宣白承氣湯 Gypsum and Rhubarb Combination)	
	Lung fever moves to the intestine	Diarrhea with yellow stool	Quick	Yellow fur	Cleanse fever, stop diarrhea	*Ko-ken-chin-lien-tang* (葛根芩連湯 Pueraria, Coptis and Scute Combination) *Ko-ken-tang* (葛根湯 Pueraria Combination)	
Ying and *hsueh*		Spiritual vexation, delirium, or maculation, or aggitation of blood	Thin	Dark red	Refer to spring-feverish disease below		

Table 9. Comparison of *Wei*, *Ch'i*, *Ying*, and *Hsueh* Stage of Spring-feverish Disease

Stage		Conformation			Treatment		
		Chief symptoms	Pulse	Tongue	Rule	Indicated formulas	Formula modification
Wei		Chillphobia, anhidrosis, somatic fever, thirst, vexation in heart, turbid yellow urine	Floating, quick	Thin-white fur with red substrate	Disperse surface, cleanse interior	*Tsung-shih-chieh-keng-tang* (葱豉桔梗湯 Allium and Platycodon Combination)	If internal fever is strong, scute may be added
Ch'i	Evils stagnated at lesser yang meridian	Alternating chills and fever, bitter mouth, hypochondrial pain, thoracic depression, tendency to vomit	Chordal, quick	Thin, greasy fur	Cleanse and discharge lesser yang	*Hsiao-chai-hu-tang* (小柴胡湯 Minor Bupleurum Combination) *Hao-chin-ching-tan-tang* (蒿芩清膽湯 Ching-hao and Scute Combination)	
	Outbreak at sunlight yang meridian	Strong fever, thirst, vexation in heart, perspiration	Surging, big	Arid tongue, yellow fur	Use acrid-chilly herbs to cleanse *ch'i*	*Pai-hu-tang* (白虎湯 Gypsum Combination)	For injury of *ch'i* and yin, ginseng is added.
	Fever trapped in stomach	Tidal fever, delirium, constipation, bound fever flowing elsewhere	Submerged, forceful	Arid tongue, yellow fur	Discharge firmness in luminal viscera	*Tiao-wei-cheng-ch'i-tang* (調胃承氣湯 Rhubarb and Mirabilitum Combination)	For dried-up fluids, give *Tseng-yeh-cheng-chi-teng* (增液承氣湯)

Table 9. Continued

Stage		Conformation			Treatment		
		Chief symptoms	Pulse	Tongue	Rule	Indicated formulas	Formula modification
Ying		Somatic fever, spiritual vexation, restless sleep at night, mild thirst, or unconsciousness with delirium	Thin, quick	Dry, dark red	Cleanse *ying* and discharge fever	*Niu-huang-ching-hsin-wan*,[1] *Ching-ying-tang*[2] associated with *An-kung-niu-huang-wan*[3]	In presence of maculation, add a little *Hua-pan-tang* (化斑湯 Gypsum and Oryza Combination) in case of wind agitation, add gambir, scorpion, etc.
Hsueh	Feverish blood flows randomly	Hematemesis, epistaxis, bloody stool, unconsciousness, delirium	Thin, quick	Dry, dark red	Cool blood and detoxify toxin	*Hsi-chiao-ti-huang-tang*,[4] *Chih-pao-tan*,[5] *Huang-lien-ah-chiao-tang*[6]	
	Yin weakness with thriving fire	Vexation in heart, inability to lie down	Thin, quick	Dark red tongue or yellow fur	Cleanse fever, nourish yin	*Hsi-chiao-ti-huang-tang*,[4] *Huang-lien-ah-chiao-tang*[6]	
	Weakness, wind agitates internally	Lethargy, spasms and flaccidity, more fever on palms and soles than on backs of hands and feet, digital vemication, or simultaneous appearance of faint and retching	Thin, quick, forceless	Dry, dark red tongue without saliva	Nourish yin, extinguish wind	*Ti-huang-yin-tzu*, *Chia-chien-fu-mo-tang*[8]	

1 *Niu-huang-ching-hsin-wan* (牛黃淸心丸 Bos and Musk Formula)
2 *Ching-ying-tang* (淸營湯 Rhinoceros and Scrophularia Combination)
3 *An-kung-niu-huang-wan* (安宮牛黃丸Bos and Curcuma Formula)
4 *Hsi-chiao-ti-huang-tang* (犀角地黃湯Rhinoceros and Rehmannia Combination)
5 *Chih-pao-tan* (至寶丹Rhinoceros and Succinum Formula)
6 *Huang-lien-ah-chiao-tang* (黃連阿膠湯Coptis and Gelatin Combination)
7 *Ti-huang-yin-tzu* (地黃飲子 Rehmannia Combination)
8 *Chia-chien-fu-mo-tang* (加減復脈湯 Baked Licorice Combination modified)

Table 10. Comparison of *Wei, Ch'i, Ying,* and *Hsueh* Stages of Summer-feverish Disease

Disease stage		Conformation			Treatment		
		Chief symptoms	Pulse	Tongue fur	Rule	Indicated formulas	Formula modifications
Wei		Headache, generalized fever, anhidrosis, chillphobia, body spasms, vexation in heart, depression in stomach area		Thin, greasy	Disperse and drive out summer heat and moisture	*Hsiang-ju-yin* (香薷飲 Elsholtzia Combination) with lonicera and forsythia	For external chill, add *San-wu-hsiang-ju-yin* (三物香薷飲 Elsholtzia Combination). For internal fever, add *Huang-lien-hsiang-ju-yin* (黃連香薷飲 Coptis and Elsholtzia Combination)
Ch'i	Fever, scorching sunlight yang	Strong fever, annoying thirst, perspiration, labored breathing	Surging, big	Yellow	Cleanse summer heat, preserve fluids	*Pai-hu-tang* (白虎湯 Gypsum Combination)	For accompaniment by moisture, add atractylodes for injuries of *ch'i* and yin, add ginseng
	Alternate blockage by summer heat and moisture	Somatic fever, perspiration without resolution of symptoms, depression and vexation tending to cause vomiting and red urine	Soft, quick	Greasy	Discharge fever, resolve moisture	*San-shih-tang* (三石湯 Talc, Calcite, and Gypsum Combination) *Pai-hu-tang* (白虎湯 Gypsum Combination)	

Table 10. Continued

Disease stage	Conformation			Treatment		
	Chief symptoms	Pulse	Tongue fur	Rule	Indicated formulas	Formula modifications
Ying	Cardiac vexation, disturbed sleep, delirium	Empty, quick	Red to dark red	Cleanse *ying*, open up cavities	*Ching-ying-tang* (清營湯 Rhinoceros and Scrophularia Combination) *Tzu-hsueh-tan* (紫雪丹Rhinoceros and Antelope Horn Formula)	
Hsueh	Scorching fever, vexation, irritation, hematemesis, epistaxis	Thin, quick	Dark red	Cool blood, unblock obstructions	*Hsi-chiao-ti-huang-tang* (犀角地黃湯 Rhinoceros and Rehmannia Combination) *Shen-hsi-tan* (神犀丹 Rhinoceros and Lonicera Formula)	In case of maculation, add scrophularia, forsythia seed core, *jen-chung-huang* (prepared licorice), leaves of small-leaf isatis

Table 11. Comparison of Summer-faint, Summer-wind, Summer-phthisis, and Summer-filth Diseases

Disease type	Chief symptoms	Treatment rule	Indicated formulas
Summer-faint	Sudden fainting, chilling limbs, dirty face, arid teeth	Cleanse heart, open up cavities	*Niu-huang-ching-hsin-wan* (牛黃淸心丸 Bos and Musk Formula), *Tzu-hsueh-tan* (紫雲丹 Rhinoceros and Antelope Horn Formula), *Ching-ying-tang* (淸營湯 Rhinoceros and Scrophularia Combination), *An-kung-niu-huang-wan* (安宮牛黃丸 Bos and Curcuma Formula)
Summer-wind	Sudden fainting, convulsions	Cleanse fever, extinguish wind	*Ling-yang-kou-teng-tang* (羚羊鈎藤湯 Antelope Horn and Gambir Combination) in conjunction with *Tzu-hsueh-tan* (紫雪丹Rhinoceros and Antelope Horn Formula) or *Chih-pao-tan* (至寶丹 Rhinoceros and Succinum Formula)
Summer-phthisis	Annoying fever, hemoptysis asthma	Cool blood, cleanse lungs	*Chu-shu-tiao-yuan-fa* (袪暑調元法 Gypsum and Hoelen Combination) in conjunction with *Ching-lo-yin* (淸絡飮 Lonicera and Lotus Leaf Combination)
Summer-filth	Vexation, depression, nausea, vomiting, fainting	Dispel filth with fragrant herbs	*Huo-hsiang-cheng-chi-san* (藿香正氣散 Agastache Formula), or with *Yu-shu-tan* (玉樞丹 Pleione and Nutgalls Formula)

Table 12. Comparison of *Wei, Ch'i, Ying,* and *Hsueh* Stages of Moisture-feverish Disease

Disease stage		Conformation			Treatment		
		Chief symptoms	Pulse	Tongue	Rule	Indicated formulas	Formula modifications
Wei		First there is mild chillphobia, then only fever without chill; perspiration, chest distention, sweet taste in mouth, thirst without desire to drink water	Soft, moderate	White, greasy fur	Disperse and resolve moisture with fragrant herbs	*Fang-hsiang-hua-cho-fa* (芳香化濁法Magnolia and Agastache Combination)	For myalgia and arthralgia, add soya bean germ, hoelen crust, tetrapanax, *tsang-chu* bark
Ch'i	When tends toward more moisture	Low body fever, fondness for hot beverages, chest depression, spiritual dullness, body heaviness	Soft, moderate	White, greasy fur	Disperse, resolve and seep off moisture	*Huo-pu-hsia-ling-tang* (藿朴夏苓湯 Agastache and Polyporus Combination), *San-jen-tang* (三仁湯 Apricot, Coix, and Cluster Combination)	For moisture obstructing clean cavities and causing spiritual dullness, add acorus, turmeric, *Yu-shu-tan* (玉樞丹Pleione and Nutgalls Formula)
	When tends toward more fever	Strong fever, bitter mouth, retching, thirst with desire to drink, cardiac vexation, chest distention, constipation, diarrhea	Soft, quick	Red tongue with yellow greasy fur	Resolve turbidity with fragrant herbs, cleanse fever, discharge moisture	*Kan-lu-hsiao-tu-tan* (甘露消毒丹 Talc and Scute Formula), *Wangs-lien-pu-yin* (王氏連朴飲 Coptis and Acorus Combination) in association with scute and talc	For constipation, use purgatives; for spiritual dullness, add *Niu-huang-ching-hsi-wan* (牛黃清心丸 Bos and Musk Formula)
Ying and *hsueh*		Spiritual dullness, limbic chilling, or hematemesis, epistaxis, bloody stool	Thin, quick	Dark red fur		Refer to spring-feverish disease	For *ch'i* prostration due to discharge of blood first give *Tu-shen-tang* (獨參湯 Ginseng Combination), then *Huang-tu-tang* (黃土湯 **Fu-lung-kan** Combination)

A. Wind feverish disease

This disease exhibits excessive surface fever in the beginning and offends the lungs first of all. The disease should not be treated with acrid-warm herbs for fear they will injure the pericardium. Treatment usually employs surface-resolving, lung-dispersing, and fever-cleansing herbs (See Table 8).

B. Spring feverish disease

This disease is commonly seen in the spring. Its treatment principally involves cleansing and discharging the internal fever (See Table 9). If a surface conformation still exists, the formula must also include surface-resolving herbs, though care must be taken in treating the drying up of humors.

C. Summer feverish disease

This disease often occurs in the summer. During the process of pathological change, injuries to the fluids and *ch'i* are observed. The rule of treatment is to cleanse summer heat and discharge fever. Moisture or chill symptoms frequently accompany summer feverish disease (See Table 10). On such occasions, moisture-dispelling or chill-dispersing herbs are added accordingly.

Other conditions belonging to this disease include summer faint, summer wind, summer phthisis, and summer filth, compared in Table 11.

D. Moisture feverish disease

This disease is caused by moisture fever evil and occurs between summer and autumn. It requires treatment by dispersing, resolving and seeping moisture or by cleansing fever and discharging moisture (See Table 12).

E. Hidden summer heat disease

This disease is caused by the evils of summer heat and moisture. It occurs after the autumn and is treated the same as summer feverish and moisture feverish diseases. Generally if there is more heat than moisture, it is treated by the method for summer feverish diseases. If there is more moisture than fever, it is treated as per moisture feverish disease. Formulas commonly used for this disease are:

1. For internal fever with surface conformation

(A) *Huang-lien-hsiang-ju-yin* (黃連香薷飲 Coptis and Elsholtzia Combination) or *Yin-chiao-san* (銀翹散 Lonicera and Forsythia Formula) treats *ch'i* stage with surface symptoms (headache, chillphobia, fever, anhidrosis, cardiac vexation, thirst, red and short urine, stomachic distention, and greasy tongue fur).

(B) *Yin-chiao-san* (銀翹散) plus raw rehmannia, moutan, red peony, and ophiopogon treats *ying* stage with surface symptoms (fever, mild chillphobia, headache, scanty sweating, dry mouth, no thirst, cardiac vexation, red tongue without fur). The formulation uses acrid and cool herbs to resolve the surface, cleanse the *ying*, and discharge fever.

2. For evils located at the lesser yang area

The symptoms exhibited are alternating chills and fever resembling malaria, thirst, vexation, stomachic distention, greasy tongue fur, somatic fever that becomes more severe in the afternoon and most severe at dusk but lessens after perspiration the next morning. The scorching fever of the chest and abdomen, however, remains constant throughout.

Treatment for this condition calls for *Hao-chin-ching-tan-tang* (蒿芩清膽湯 Ching-hao and Scute Combination) to cleanse and discharge the gallbladder of the lesser yang meridian and also to discharge moisture.

3. For fever trapped in the stomach and intestine

This disease is caused by two sets of conditions. One is the intermingling of moisture and fever which get stagnated in the stomach and intestine. The symptoms are scorching fever in the chest and abdomen; vomiting and nausea; intermittent watery diarrhea having a color resembling the soybean leaven that is used for pickling cucumbers; and greasy yellow tongue fur. *Chih-shih-tao-chih-tang* (枳實導滯湯 Chih-shih and Rhubarb Combination) is the formula frequently used to discharge fever, manage *ch'i,* resolve moisture, cleanse fever, and detoxify toxicity. The other condition is sunlight yang visceral firmness with fever occurring in the small intestine. The expressed symptoms are somatic fever; annoying thirst, abdominal distention and pain resisting pressing; short, red, and painful urination; and arid yellow sputum. *Tao-chih-cheng-chi-tang* (導赤承氣湯 Peony and Coptis Combination) purges and discharges fever in this condition.

4. For evils located in the ying and hsueh stages

This illness occurs as two types. One is fever in the heart that moves downward to the small intestine. The other is fever that closes off the pericardium, causing vascular stagnation. The former manifests fever which is mild in the daytime and severe at night, vexation causing insomnia, dry mouth, thirst without desire to drink, urine red in color and short in duration, fever with pain, and a dark red tongue. The formula commonly used for cleansing and purging purposes is *Tao-chih-ching-hsin-tang* (導赤清心湯 Rehmannia and Lophatherum Combination). The latter type exhibits fever that becomes severe at night, unconsciousness with delirium, soaking the mouth with water but not intending to drink it, a tongue that appears dry but is still moist or looks dull, purplish, and moist. *Hsi-ti-ching-lo-yin* (犀地清絡飲 Rhinoceros and Moutan Combination) is often used to cleanse the *ying* and discharge fever.

F. Autumn aridity disease

This disease is caused by the autumn aridity evil. Clinically it manifests the symptoms of dried fluids or constipation when the evil enters the intestine (See Table 13).

G. Feverish toxin

This disease generally occurs in the winter and spring as a consequence of weather abnormalities. In addition to surface

Table 13. Comparison of *Wei, Ch'i, Ying,* and *Hsueh* Stages of Autumn-Aridity Disease

Disease stage		Conformation			Treatment		
		Chief symptoms	Pulse	Tongue	Rule	Indicated formulas	Formula modifications
Wei	Cool aridity	Headache, chillphobia, anhidrosis, stuffy nose, dry pharynx, cough with thin sputum	Floating	Thin, white and dry fur	Use acrid herbs to open up cavities, and warm herbs to moisten aridity	*Hsiang-su-san* (香蘇散 Cyperus and Perilla Formula) *Hsing-su-san* (杏蘇散 Apricot Seed and Perilla Formula)	
	Warm aridity	Headache, fever, cough with scanty sputum, dry mouth, dry nose	Quick, big	Thin, white dry fur, red at apex and ridges of tongue	Use acrid, cool sweet herbs to moisten aridity	*Sang-chu-yin* (桑菊飲 Morus and Chrysanthemum Combination) plus pear skin, fritillaria, adenophora	
		Dry cough, tinnitus, ocular hyperemia, pharyngeal ache, dry mouth and tongue	Quick	Red tongue, yellow fur	Cleanse and discharge fire fever, nourish yin and moisten aridity	*Chiao-ho-tang* (翹荷湯 Forsythia and Mentha Combination) *Sha-shen-mai-tung-tang* (沙參麥	If surface evil has been resolved but there is abdominal distention and constipation, give *Wu-jen-wan*

Table 13. Continued

Disease stage	Conformation			Treatment		
	Chief symptoms	Pulse	Tongue	Rule	Indicated formulas	Formula modifications
Ch'i					冬湯 Adenophora and Ophiopogon Combination)	(五仁丸 Persica and Biota Formula) with trichosanthes and baker's garlic; if there is strong binding fever, give *Tiao-wei-cheng-chi-tang* (調胃承氣湯 Rhubarb and Mirabilitum Combination) with fresh *ho-sho-wu* and fresh raw rehmannia
Ying and *hsueh*	Unconsciousness, spasms, flaccidity of muscles	Thin, quick	Dark red		*Ching-ying-tang* (淸營湯 Rhinoceros and Scrophularia Combination)	

symptoms, it also exhibits reddening, swelling, fever and aching, or even erosion and ulceration. Its manifestations are many and equivalent to, for example, what Western medicine terms scarlet fever, mumps, measles, and diphtheria. The commonly used formula is *Pu-chi-hsiao-tu-yin* (普濟消毒飲 , Scute and Cimicifuga Combination) which causes evils to be expelled from the body and detoxifies poisons.

H. Feverish plague

This disease, characterized by a sudden onset, is grave and vicious and highly contagious. It can spread to many people quickly. In Chinese medicine, it is divided into moisture feverish plague and summer aridity plague.

(A) Moisture feverish plague. This plague is induced and caused by moisture feverish plague toxin. A lesion appears at the semi-surface/semi-internal region. The etiology is a disease evil that invades the body through the mouth and nose and stays in the stomach. It manifests itself in the following two conformations:

(1) At the onset, there is chillphobia, strong fever, and later, fever without chills. Fever occurs day and night, becoming more severe at dusk. The patient also has headache, somatic ache, a quick pulse that is neither floating nor submerged, and a dark red tongue with white fur that resembles accumulated powder. Treatment by sweating and purgation methods is generally prohibited. Commonly *Ta-yuan-yin* (達原飲 Areca Seed and Magnolia Combination) from the *Wen i lun* (温疫論 Exposition on Feverish Plague) is used to disperse and discharge toxic evils.

(2) For symptoms of strong fever, thirst, profuse sweating, yellow tongue fur, and a surging and quick pulse, *Pai-hu-tang* (白虎湯 Gypsum Combination) is used to cleanse and purge the sunlight yang fever. If the fever binds with the stomach, there will be annoying thirst and somatic fever, with additional afternoon symptoms of vexation, irritability, nostrils resembling bituminous coal, and a tongue that is blackened throughout and has spikes growing on it. This is treated with *Ta-cheng-chi-tang* (大承氣湯 Major Rhubarb Combination) or like formulas to

immediately purge the fever toxin.

(B) Summer aridity plague. This illness is due to the induction of plague toxin of summer aridity and moisture fever. This disease occurs mostly in those years when there is a long drought and fierce summer heat where pathogenic toxin is present everywhere, outside and throughout the body, and exhibits a thriving state of fever toxin. The symptoms are strong generalized fever; vexation, irritability, and uneasiness; headache; abdominal ache; vomiting; diarrhea, macules, intestinal colic causing extreme pain, and stench occurring throughout the body. Formulas used to cleanse the toxin include *Ching-wen-pai-tu-yin* (清瘟敗毒飲 Gypsum and Moutan Combination) and *Shih-chuan-ku-han-chiu-pu-tang* (十全苦寒救補湯 Gypsum and Anemarrhena Combination).

The conformations and therapeutic explanations of the feverish plague diseases are noted in Table 14.

7
Diagnosis of Feverish Diseases

Wang (diagnosis by observation), *wen* (diagnosis by olfaction and auscultation), *wun* (diagnosis by inquiry), and *chieh* (diagnosis by pulse palpation) are the four methods of diagnosis in traditional Chinese medicine. Through the four diagnostic methods, a physician gathers a wide range of pathological data and disease information which he analyzes and refines. This information directs clinical practice. It is therefore untrue to say that one can understand the etiology of a disease simply by taking the patient's pulse without referring to additional disease information. It must be noted that there are hundreds of thousands of diseases and pathological changes, but there are only twenty-eight kinds of pulses. How could a disease be assigned to a given pulse? Only by confirming the disease with the pulse and vice versa, and then simultaneously referring to both the disease and the pulse can we made a correct diagnosis. If we can proceed further by combining these diagnostic methods with the scientific ex-

Table 14. Comparison of Moisture-feverish Plague and Summer-aridity Plague Diseases

Disease type		Conformation			Treatment		
		Chief symptoms	Pulse	Tongue	Rule	Indicated formulas	Formula modifications
Moisture-feverish plague	Evils stagnated at diaphram area	Initially chillphobia and strong fever, then only fever without chill; headache, somatic ache	Neither quick, floating nor submerged	Turbid and greasy fur or like accumulated powder	Unblock, disperse, discharge, dispel toxins	*Ta-yuan-yin* (達原飲 Areca Seed and Magnolia Combination)	Suitable methods and formulas are chosen depending on whether the evil is in meridians or luminal viscera
	Evil migrates into sunlight yang area	Strong fever, thirst, distention and aching at chest-diaphragm area; or constipation with delirium	Surging-quick, or submerged-quick	Coarse, parched, yellow or black fur	Use cool herbs to resolve internal fever, or save yin, and unblock luminal viscera	*Pai-hu-tang* (白虎湯 Gypsum Combination) *Ta-yuan-yin* (達原飲) excluding Chinese cardamon and including rhubarb. *Ta-cheng-chi-tang* (大承氣湯 Major Rhubarb Combination)	
	Evil fire flaring internally in *ying* and *hsueh* stages	Purplish-black macules, irritability, thirst and crazy utterances	Surging, big and quick	Dark red tongue with parched, yellow or black fur	Cleanse both blood and *ch'i*, resolve macules, and detoxify toxin	*Hsi-chiao-ti-huang-tang* (犀角地黄湯 Rhinoceros and Rehmannia Combination) *Hua-pan-tang* (化斑湯 Gypsum and Oryza Combination) plus *Huang-lien-chieh-tu-tang* (黄連解毒湯	

Table 14. Continued

Disease type		Conformation			Treatment		
		Chief symptoms	Pulse	Tongue	Rule	Indicated formulas	Formula modifications
						Coptis and Scute Combination)	
Summer-aridity plague	Activated type	Chillphobia, fever, severe headache (as if the head has been cut by an axe), blurred vision in both eyes, annoying arthralgia; even irritating thirst, delirium, unconsciousness, hematemesis, and epistaxis	Submerged, quick	Arid tongue, yellow fur	Use acrid, cool herbs at high doses to cleanse fever and detoxify toxin	*Ching-wen-pai-tu-yin* (淸瘟敗毒飲 Gypsum and Moutan Combination) *Wu-chih-yin* (五汁飲 Pear Five Juice Combination)	
	Depressed type	Greenish-purple facial complexion, or like micaceous earth, adverse limbic chilling, head sweats (like raining), headache like head is cut up, lumbago, tendency to vomit but cannot, tendency to have diarrhea but cannot pass stools	Six types of pulses are thin, and submerged, like a hidden pulse	Arid tongue, yellow fur	Use acrid, cool herbs at high doses to cleanse fever and detoxify toxin	*Ching-wen-pai-tu-yin* (淸瘟敗毒飲) plus *Tzu-hsueh-tan* (紫雪丹 Rhinoceros and Antelope Horn Formula) *Chih-pao-tan* (至寶丹 Rhinoceros and Succinum Formula)	

amination methods of modern medicine, we can then make an unmistakably correct diagnosis.

The commonly used methods for examining and diagnosing feverish diseases are these:

A. Observation

Observation occupies a very important position in the diagnosis of disease. The *Nan ching* (Classic of Medical Difficulties) says, "To get the disease information by observation is known as 'divinity'." Because conditions inside the body reflect on the outside, a physician proficient in the diagnosis by observation can see at once the disease information and can tell whether it is a grave or mild, a chronic or new disease, and can make a prognosis without referring to the pulse diagnosis.

If we combine the information from observing, taking the pulse and a disease history inquiry, and confirm each diagnosis with the others, we will not miss any information. Furthermore, if we make use of present-day roentgenoscopy, it will be even more helpful.

1. Complexion

The chapter on treatment of fever with acupuncture in the *Nei ching* says, "If there is fever in the liver, the left cheek becomes red first of all; fever in the lungs, the right cheek; fever in the heart, the face; fever in the spleen, the nose; fever in the kidneys, the chin."

Most feverish diseases manifest a red as well as a filthy and dull face. This is because the fever evil steams upward to cause fluids to well up over the face, hence the face becomes red, filthy, and dull. In such a face, if the end of the nose appears bright and glossy, the condition is favorable; if the nose end is withered and arid, the condition is critical. If both the face and the eyes are red, it indicates a thriving fever of the sunlight yang. It is the fever that scorches the lungs' yin and causes conjunctival hyperemia. Since the white parts of the eyes belong to the lungs, lung fever is reflected externally in this part. After recovery from a feverish disease, a slightly red face, a quick pulse, and fever in the evening indicate weakened gastric yin.

After recovery from a feverish disease, a dull yellow facial complexion together with a soft and weak pulse indicates splenic weakness.

After recovery from a feverish disease, a pale facial complexion and a thin-weak pulse indicate the yin injury has involved the yang, and there are deficiencies in blood and *ch'i.*

2. Eyes

The chapter on great perplexities in the *Ling shu* volume of the *Nei ching* says, "The essential vitality of the five solid viscera and the six hollow viscera flows to the eyes and becomes the pupils." The shine of vigor exists in the eyes. If the eyes discharge excreta and tears yet shine vigorously, we say the eyes have the shine of vigor. If the eyes do not discharge excreta and tears, the white portion appears dark and turbid, the black portion appears dull and dim and without luster, and the shine appears loose, diffuse, and superficial, the eyes are said to be without the shine of vigor. A patient with the shine of vigor in his eyes is in a favorable condition, one without is unfavorable. A patient who opens his eyes because he wants to see people has a yang conformation. One who closes his eyes because he does not want to see people has a yin conformation. (On some occasions in which the patient closes his eyes because of photophobia, it is a condition of yin weakness and internal fever.)

If at the beginning of a feverish disease the inner canthi of both eyes are red, it signals an internal fever conformation. Blood fever also exhibits itself in red eyes. Yellow sclera and ulcerous canthi indicate moisture fever. Unclear eyes and pupils and pupils that have trouble are due to a fever evil steaming upward. Blurred vision and unconsciousness indicate fever entering the pericardium. A fixed straight stare or strabismus results from hepatic wind moving internally. If the shine of the pupils becomes diffuse and scattered, the fever has entered the brain, and it is a dangerous conformation. Since the eye tract connects with the brain in the upper part of the body, the brain is the sea of marrow and the essence of the marrow is the pupils, scattering, diffusing or shrinking of the pupils' shine of vigor reflects pathological changes of the brain and marrow.

3. *Nose*

The nose is the opening of the lungs and belongs to the spleen meridian. If the nose exhibits a bright moist color, it indicates the disease is healing; a green color indicates the liver *ch'i* is stagnated or there is anoxia; a black color denotes water vapor; a white color reflects *ch'i* weakness; a red color signals lung fever; and a yellow color portends moisture fever.

Stuffy nose, sniveling, or dry nostrils are symptoms of contracting external winds and fever. If the snivel is thin and clean, it is contracting of external winds and chills. If the snivel is turbid with a fishy odor, it is a *pi yuan* (ozena) condition due to fever stagnated in the lungs.

If the nostrils are as black as bituminous coal, it indicates the fever has injured the lungs, the fever being caused by yang toxin which has penetrated deeply. This leads to a critical condition in most cases. If the nasal alae wave and the patient breathes with difficulty, it portends that the lung *ch'i* is going to be exhausted. The pulse in such cases must be quick and rushing but forceless upon pressing. Chinese herbs alone are not enough to ensure a prompt cure. Oxygen inhalation, even tracheotomy and artificial respiration should be performed. Chinese formulas such as *Sheng-mo-san* (生脈散 Ginseng, Schizandra, and Ophiopogon Formula) may be given to astringe the pulmonary *ch'i*. Using both Chinese and Western therapeutic methods, many lives can be saved. Sometimes stagnation and obstruction of sputum fever also manifest a chordal, slippery, and quick pulse or a submerged and quick one.

4. *Mouth*

The mouth is the opening for the spleen. The spleen and the stomach have an internal-surface relationship to each other. By diagnosing the lips and oral cavity we can detect the pathological changes of the spleen and stomach.

If both the mouth and the lips are red, it indicates splenic and stomachic fever. A dark red color is a sign of a firm fever. A dark red color with a dry, parched state indicates thriving fever injuring body fluids.

Dark lips and mouth portend anoxia. If there is blackening around the mouth, the mouth shapes like a fish's, and the patient only exhales but doesn't inhale, it is an extremely critical symptom.

5. *Ears*

The kidneys have the ears as their openings. The ears belong to the lesser yang meridian because the lesser yang meridian transversely shunts the inside of the ears. Ear diseases such as deafness and swelling and aching of the ears are due to wind fever in the lesser yang meridian. In feverish diseases, deafness is due to an up-flushing of the fever evil.

If the ears are thick, fleshy, moist and glossy, the condition is mild even though the patient has a disease. If the ears are thin, fleshless, dry and withered, it indicates a renal yin deficiency. Dry, withered, parched, and blackened ears indicate fever scorching the renal yin that causes extreme depletion of renal water. Redness in the body of the ear signals internal fever. Shrunken or atrophied ear bodies indicate exhaustion of renal *ch'i,* which is difficult to cure in most cases.

6. *Tongue*

Diagnosis of the tongue includes both the tongue texture and fur. The tongue texture was known as *she pen* in ancient times. Chang Hsu-ku (章虛谷) of the Ching (清) dynasty said, "By observing the tongue texture we can detect yin, yang, weakness, and firmness. By inspecting the tongue fur and fur filth, we can see whether the evil is chill, fever, weak or firm." In the *I men pang ho* (醫門棒喝), tongue diagnosis is of great significance to feverish diseases. Symptoms commonly seen with the tongue texture and fur in feverish diseases are:

(a) Shape: A normal person's tongue body is soft, pliable, brisk, and sensitive. Under the high fever of a feverish disease, the following symptoms often will appear.

i) Stiffened: It will have a dark red texture, accompanied by unconsciousness and delirium, due to fever intruding into the pericardium. As fire fever injures the secretion of fluids, the tongue body becomes stiff, and the patient has difficulty and harshness in speaking.

ii) Agitative: The tongue agitates in the mouth, extending and retracting, shaking, moving up and down and to the left and right, like the licking action of a snake's tongue. It is due to a thriving fever in the heart meridian, and a liver wind that moves internally.

iii) Trembling: The tongue body trembles ceaselessly when the tongue extends out. If this occurs while the evil fever is thriving, the tongue will be dark red and trembling, due to culminant fever generating wind. In the late stage of a feverish disease, if the tongue appears pale-colored, and moves slowly and mildly, it is due to a weakness in both the heart and the spleen.

iv) Curled, shortened: The tongue is incapable of extending. It even contracts to form a mass. The cause is a culminant fever causing a movement of wind, and sputum obstructing at the tongue root. At times, it is also due to ignorance in the use of purging treatments, which lead to a curling and shortening of the tongue, black arid tongue fur with spikes, and dried-up fluids.

v) Swollen: The tongue is bright red and extends out of the mouth but can't retract. This is due to extreme fever in the cardiac meridian. If the tongue is swollen but incapable of extending out of the mouth, and the lips are also slightly swollen, it is due to splenic moistness, stomachic fever, and a flushing-up of toxic fever.

(b) Color: A normal person's tongue is pink. The tongue is frisky, moist, and lustrous. It is sufficiently supplied with blood, is soft and tender, and moves freely. As the fever evil enters the *ying* system, the tongue will definitely become dark red.

i) Dark red: The *Wen je lun* (温熱論) says, "As the fever enters the *ying* stage, the tongue color will definitely become dark red. A purely dark red tongue that appears fresh and lustrous is an indication that the evil has left the *wei* and entered the *ying* and that fever is at the pericardium. A dark, red and dry tongue indicates fire evil robbing the *ying*, and stomachic aridity injuring the fluids. If at the beginning the tongue is dark red and has yellow-white fur, it indicates that evil at the *ch'i* stage has not been completely depleted and has entered the *ying* stage.

If the tongue is only red but not dark red at the edge, yellowish white at the center, and the patient feels thirsty, it indicates the fever is not in the blood domain but in the *ch'i* domain of the upper warmer where the *ch'i* fever scorches fluids. If the tongue is dark red and the upper surface is sticky and has a greasy-looking fur, it indicates obstruction and accumulation of turbid dirt in the middle warmer. If only the central line of the tongue is dark red, it indicates a gastric fever whereby the heart and the *ying* are injured. Up-flaring of cardiac fire that causes a tender and red tongue is a weakness fever. A pale red and dry tongue indicates injured gastric fluids, and *ch'i* (vapor) not transformed into fluids. This kind of tongue is often observed at the late stage of feverish diseases.

ii) Red with red spots: Large red spots scattered on a red tongue indicate toxic fever invading the heart and entering the blood domain with a tendency toward maculation.

iii) Red with black spots: Black spots scattered on a red tongue indicate a feverish fever has entered the sunlight yang stage and red macules are going to erupt on the body.

iv) Strawberry (also known as wild raspberry): The upper surface of the tongue is bright red, and all papillae are exposed like a strawberry. This is a characteristic symptom of scarlet fever, which is also an indication of fever entering the *ying* and blood stages.

v) Bright red and eroding (like being peeled): In this condition, toxic fever has entered the blood stage. This is often accompanied by bleeding symptoms such as hematemesis, bloody stool, and hypodermal bleeding. This kind of tongue is often present in what Western medicine terms "diffusive intravascular coagulation". The tongue aches severely upon eating, hindering swallowing. It is also a dangerous symptom.

vi) Mirror surface: The tongue appears dark red and glossy like a kidney. It is due to depletion and exhaustion of gastric yang, and difficult to cure.

(c) Fur: A normal person's tongue fur is neither thick nor greasy, but thin and evenly distributed, or slightly thicker at the middle and root areas, and is of a suitable degree of moistness. Chang Hsu-ku (章虛谷) of the Ching (清) dynasty said, "The spleen and stomach are critical to the body. When evils enter the stomach, fur occurs, just like grass growing on the ground. In healthy individuals, slight thin fur is often present which is likened to grass roots and signifies gastric vitality. If the tongue appears glossy like a mirror, it is without enlivening vitality, and is likened to a grassless soil which has become depleted. When a stomach with vitality is invaded by evils, tongue fur thickens just like grass growing higher upon addition of good soil. Hence, tongue fur can be used to detect the weakness, firmness, chill, or fever of a disease, or the depth of intrusion and intensity of an evil." (Please see *I men pang ho* 醫門棒喝 for the above quotation). This explains how observing tongue fur enables us to tell the state of gastric vitality. In case of stronger turbid *ch'i* in the gastro-intestinal tract the tongue fur will definitely be thick. By "turbid *ch'i*" we mean either the stagnated foods and beverages or accumulated moisture and sputum. As the fur turns from thick to thin, it signifies a retreating of evils and a healing of the disease. As the fur turns from thin to thick, it indicates the evils are getting exhuberant and the disease advances to a worse condition. If on a tongue formerly covered with a thick layer of fur throughout, the fur subsides rapidly and the tongue becomes glossy and bright without saliva, it portends that the gastric *ch'i* is going to be exhausted, an extremely dangerous symptom.

The color changes of tongue fur are divided into white, yellow, and black as described below:

i) White: The tongue is pink and covered with a thin layer of white fur. This normal thin white fur is also present at the beginning of feverish diseases, but the tongue must then be red which indicates the evil is not yet deep in the body but only at the *wei* stage. A tongue fur with both yellow and white colors indicates the external evil has not been resolved yet, and it has moved gradually inward. A grey and white fur and absence of thirst signifies moisture sputum and unconverted yang *ch'i* in most cases. The presence of a white, sticky, greasy fur, bitter mouth, and thirst indicates that moisture evil has been transformed into fever. If the condition of the oral cavity is normal but there is not thirst, it is because moisture is gradually turning into fever. If tongue fur is white, thick, and dry, it signals injured gastric fluid although the disease evil has not yet penetrated deeply. A white, thin, dry fur indicates the lung fluid is injured. A white, greasy fur with a dark red substrate signifies suppressed moisture and hidden fever. If a white fur resembles accumulated powder spreading all over the tongue surface and the tongue edge is dark purplish-red, it is known as a *pai sha she* (white sandy tongue) which reflects internally bound fever toxin, coagulated and accumulated dirts, and turbid substances. When the ancients said white tongue fur stands for a chill conformation, they referred to a condition in which the fur must be white but not dry; the mouth is normal without thirst; the tongue color is pink instead of red; the abdomen is distended but not firm to pressing. Only when these symptomatic terms are fulfilled is the condition one of chilly moisture. It can be treated with such herbs as can resolve chills and dry up moisture—warm, arid drugs. In feverish diseases, although white fur is observed, the tongue must be dark red, or there must be a bitter and greasy mouth. Warm and arid drugs are contraindicated under such conditions.

ii) Yellow: Yellow fur that is slippery but not very thick is derived from white fur, and is going to be converted into fever that enters the interior. A yellow, thin and dry fur results from an external contraction which, being converted into fever, has just entered the interior in the form of gastric fever to injure fluid there. In the late stage when the evil has gone; the fluids are injured; and the fur is yellow, thick and dry, it is a sign of firm internal fever. Furthermore, if spikes grow on the tongue, the firm fever has become more severe. Furs of old yellow or greyish yellow color also belong to firm fever. All of the above-mentioned yellow furs must have a ground to support the yellow just like newly grown grass must have roots to maintain its growth. Hence, purging treatment can be used for these furs. However, if the yellow fur is glossy, slippery, and rootless, it is surface filth which can be readily scraped off, and such fur indicates intangible moisture fever and absence of gastric firm fever which should not be purged erroneously.

iii) Black: Black fur is differentiated into four types—weakness, firmness, chill, and fever. However, black fur observed in feverish diseases is only of fever and never of chill type. A black, arid and thick fur and a tongue with a red edge indicate culminant fever and dried fluids. A black fur that is arid, has spikes on it, and feels touchy to the hand is a critical symptom of culminant fever. A white fur with a growing black color at the center indicates the fever evil has moved into the interior. A red fur with a growing black center signifies a feverish disease fever has moved into the interior, is becoming critical, and is difficult to treat in most cases. If the tongue has dry black fur at the root but not at the center, it indicates a fever situated in the lower warmer. Black and dry tongue fur which is thick at the center reflects gastric aridity and yang exhaustion.

Ancient books often took black fur for a weakness chill. For such a diagnosis the black fur must be moist and slippery or very thin, or as black as bituminous coal and in no kind of black furs should the tongue color be purplish red; otherwise it is not a weakness chill. Nevertheless, it is very common that some alcoholics with bound and stagnant moisture and sputum often exhibit black moist fur on a normal tongue body. Such fur is not regarded as pathological. Very frequently a yellow brown or black fur has a connection with smoking or ingestion of colored foods. For example, eating fruits like pomegranate turns tongue fur black, whereas eating loquats produces a yellow color.

The aforementioned types of fur are those more commonly observed in feverish diseases. Since the tongue texture and tongue fur are interrelated they should be jointly observed: for example, a red tongue with white fur, a red tongue with yellow fur, a pale tongue with white fur, a pale tongue with yellow fur. These are yellow or white furs, yet different tongue colors reflect different conformations. No matter what kind of fur exists, if there are spikes growing in the fur, it is a symptom of a thriving fever.

7. Teeth

The teeth indicate the state of the bones and reflect the kidneys. The chapter on *Wu wei* (Five Tastes and Odors) in the *Ling shu* (靈樞 Spiritual Pivot) says, "The teeth are where the bones begin." The technique of diagnosing disease by observing the teeth was scarcely mentioned in ancient texts. Yeh Tien-shih (葉天士) developed this method in his *Wen je lun* (温熱論),

in which he divided the dental symptoms into the following six types: pattern formation, aridity, gnashing, filth, bleeding, and scorch.

i) Pattern formation: The teeth are indicators of the kidneys, and the gingiva is connected with a transverse branch of the gastric meridian. If the fever evil does not dry up the gastric fluids, it will exhaust the renal fluids. Blood from both meridians goes through the same area; hence as the disease condition becomes more severe, blood is disturbed, causing pattern formation on the gingiva. If the pattern is formed by yang blood, the gingiva will definitely be purple like a dry varnish; if the pattern is formed by yin blood, the color will definitely be yellow like pickled beans. In the presence of yang blood, the essential treatment is to stabilize the stomach; in the presence of yin blood, it is necessary to save the kidneys. In any case, the presence of a pickled bean color is always a dangerous sign.

ii) Aridity: If the teeth are as bright and arid as stone, gastric fever is strong. If the patient has chillphobia but no perspiration, he has a partially thriving condition in his *wei* system and requires acrid and cool herbs to discharge the *wei* and to bring about perspiration as the principal treatment. If the teeth look like withered bones, the renal fluids are dried and the condition proves difficult to cure. If the upper halves of the teeth are moist, it indicates water does not reach the upper part, the heart fire flares up, and the condition requires prompt treatment by cleaning the heart and saving water until the arid part turns moist.

iii) Gnashing: If the patient simply gnashes, it indicates gastric fever is circulating the transverse branch of the gastric meridian. (Renal fever also causes gnashing). If in addition to gnashing, the pulse and conformation also indicate degeneration, it signifies the stomach is weak and empty, and has no supply of cereals to nourish the *jon* (榮 viscera). Emptiness likes being filled up. If the tongue body does not contract but stiffens and the teeth are tightly locked and hard to open up, the condition must be either wind sputum blocking a transverse branch of the meridian or a presymptom of convulsions.

iv) Filth: Dental filth that resembles grey rice cake indicates the stomach *ch'i* is forceless, fluids are depleted, and moisture and turbidity are working their ways through the body. The condition is lethal in most cases.

v) Bleeding: If the teeth ache, clear blood flowing between teeth signifies gastric fire flaring up. If the teeth do not ache, the ministerial fire is burning internally.

vi) Scorch: Dental scorch without dental filth is a lethal sign. Dental scorch with dental filth indicates renal fever depleting gastric fluids.

B. Olfaction and Auscultation

1. Discrimination of smells

At a high fever in a feverish or fever disease, fever evil steams and fumigates from the interior toward the outside, producing a "fever odor", an abnormal smell that is detectable all over the bed in mild cases or through the whole bedroom in severe cases. Hyperhidrosis also produces a sour stench. Dirty, turbid mouth odor is often due to a gastric firm fever that flushes up. A foul odor to the stool arises from gastrointestinal firm fever, while a sour odor is due to food stagnation.

2. Discrimination of sounds and voices

Clear, loud voices with a lucid spirit are often associated with a mild condition even in the presence of high fever.

Disorderly speech indicates that fever evil has entered the interior, and the patient is going to become unconscious. Coarse, loud, or rapid breathing indicates the fever evil has invaded the lungs and the lungs are losing their normal function.

C. Inquiry

The chapter *Shih chuan* (Teacher's Instructions) in the *Ling shu* volume (靈樞·師傳篇) of the *Nei ching* (內經) states, "In clinical inquiry into the patient's defecation condition, heatstroke with polydipsia exhibits chill stool; whereas, chillstroke exhibits feverish stool." This tells us that by inquiry we can see the feverish or chilly nature of diseases. This diagnostic method stands out as the most important among the four methods. Because without inquiry we can not know the patient's subjective feeling, his anamnesis, the duration of the disease, dietary factors, occupation, living environment, etc.

Chang Ching-yueh (張景岳) of the Ming (明) dynasty summarized the essential points of diagnosis by inquiry in his *Shih wen pien* (十問篇 Ten Inquiries):

> "First inquire about chills and fevers; second, inquire about sweat; third, inquire about the head and body; fourth, inquire about urination and bowel movement; fifth, inquire about eating and drinking; sixth, inquire about chest; seventh, inquire about hearing; eighth, inquire about thirst; ninth, inquire into yin and yang by referring to pulse and complexion information; and tenth, inquire to confirm smells and spiritual state."

Chen Hsiu-yuan (陳修園) of the Ching (清) dynasty deleted the last two inquires and modified it into:

> "The ninth inquiry is about anamnesis; the tenth inquiry about the cause; then combine this information with that drawn from the patient's pathological changes after medication. In women we should also inquire about the menstrual cycle, whether it is early or late, and whether there is amenorrhea or metrorrhagia. For children, attention must also be called to smallpox and measles."

In making the diagnosis, we should grasp the important points on which to base our conformational identification. These points are described as follows.

1. Pyrexia

In feverish diseases pyrexia is divided into surface and internal fever. In surface fever, mild chillphobia at the beginning is followed by a fever without chill, thermophobia, yet thirst, and spontaneous perspiration. These symptoms of a sunlight yang conformation exhibit a quick pulse that is neither floating nor submerged. The pulse at the *chun* site is definitely bigger than at the *kuan* and *chih* sites. Fever is on the skin and exhibits a scorching feeling to the touch which lessens with prolonged touching. Fever without sweating belongs to a condition in which the evil is at the *wei* stage. It requires acrid and cool herbs to resolve the surface and drive the evil out through the surface. Modified *Sang-chu-yin* (桑菊飲 Morus and Chrysanthemum Combination) is the formula to be used. In the winter if chillphobia is stronger, add a small quantity of schizonepeta and siler or perilla leaves to dispel the surface chill. In case of strong generalized fever, spontaneous perspiration, and total absence of chillphobia, the evil has entered the *ch'i* stage, and the pulse is then slippery, big, and quick. The condition requires treatment with modified *Pai-hu-tang* (加減白虎湯).

Internal fever reflects internal binding of feverish disease fever, and firmness of the stomach. In pyrexia or tidal fever the fever begins mild but becomes stronger as pressing continues, especially of the abdomen where the fever is higher than that of the legs. Or there is limbic perspiration; abdominal distention; aching that increases when pressed; dry, hard stool; diarrhea accompanying fever; scant, red urine; even polydipsia and delirium. The pulse is mostly slippery and quick, or submerged, quick, and forceful, and bigger at the *kuan* and *chih* sites than at the *chun* site on both wrists. This condition requires immediate purgation with either of the three purgative formulas (三承氣湯 Major Rhubarb Combination, Minor Rhubarb Combination, Rhubarb and Mirabilitum Combination), *San-huang-hsieh-hsin-tang* (三黃瀉心湯 Coptis and Rhubarb Combination), or *Liang-ke-san* (涼膈散 Forsythia and Rhubarb Formula). However, because pyrexia in feverish or fever disease is often of a mixed surface-interior type, both surface-resolving and interior-attacking can be conducted at the same time. *Tseng-shun-shuang-chieh-san* (增損雙解散 Siler and Mentha Formula modified) and *Chia-wei-liang-ke-san* (加味涼膈散 Forsythia and Rhubarb Formula modified), which resolve both the surface and interior, can be used.

If the pyrexia remains unsubsided after treatment with surface-resolving and interior-attacking drugs, the problem is due to a commingling of wind chill and feverish disease fever which combine to develop into a fever toxin that constricts the muscles and skin surface. It can be treated by the toxin-extraction method using the following formula:

Castor seeds (with seed coats removed) 30g, and *Cirsium spicatum* (the fresh article is best) 120g. Pick out the cirsium stalks and discard. Boil the cirsium, take out the dregs, wipe dry, and pound the dregs together with the castor seeds into a paste. Rub the paste onto the precordium and a site on the back opposite the heart, and the bending sites of the limbs until the skin appears reddish. The next day, red measles will erupt on the rubbed sites, and the fever will recede. Here castor seeds act to extract toxins and *Cirsium spicatum* cools the blood, detoxifies, and causes the fever toxin that blocks the surface to be driven out of the body. The formula has the advantages of being cheap, convenient to apply, and efficacious. Forty years ago a patient came to me who had had unsubsided fever for many days. I rubbed him with this formula. The next day, white vesicles as large as grapes erupted on the rubbed sites, and the fever subsided a little. I again applied the formula to other body areas that had not been rubbed. Vesicles appeared on each area rubbed. Nearly the entire upper body had been rubbed before the fever finally subsided. The fever was of the plague toxin type. Several decades later, I encountered another case; this person was also cured by an application of this formula, in this case just once after red measles erupted and fever subsided.

2. Chillphobia

Chillphobia in feverish diseases often occurs at the beginning. At first it is mild chillphobia, then pyrexia without chillphobia. When it is chill, the patient feels only chill but no fever. When it is pyrexia, the patient feels only fever but no chill. This mode of chillphobia is different from that exhibited in wind chill. In a wind chill disease, chillphobia and pyrexia occur simultaneously. Chillphobia is more severe in wind chill than in feverish disease. In wind chill, the pulse is not quick, there is no thirst, and the patient will certainly have headache, generalized aches, or spasms. The condition should be treated with acrid, warm herbs to resolve the surface. The representative formulas are *Ching-fang-chieh-tu-yin* (荆防解毒飲 Schizonepeta, Siler, and Chiang-huo Combination), and *Chia-chien-chiu-wei-chiang-huo-tang* (加減九味羌活湯 Chiang-huo Combination modified). In feverish disease, there is chillphobia, quick pulse, thirst, red urine, and headache; generalized spasms rarely occur. It requires acrid, cool herbs to resolve the surface. Although there is chillphobia, acrid, warm herbs are prohibited for feverish disease. The representative formulas for this condition are modifications of *Yin-chiao-san* (銀翹散 Lonicera and Forsythia Formula).

Diseases with pyrexia and chillphobia are divided into internal injury and external contraction, which Li Tung-yuan (李東垣) of the Yuan (元) dynasty described in fine detail.

Wang Ken-tang (王肯堂) of the Ming (明) dynasty said:

> "Very few diseases have no pyrexia, and the pyrexia mode is the chief distinction between internal injury and external contracting. If the carotid pulse is bigger than the wrist pulse, it is an external contraction. If the wrist pulse is bigger than the carotid pulse, it is an internal injury. In external contraction chilling and pyrexia occur simultaneously while in internal injury, chill and fever occur alternately. Chillphobia in external contraction can't be removed even by keeping the body near a strong fire; whereas, in internal injury, chillphobia is resolved the moment the body gets warmth. A person with externally contracted chillphobia does not fear any kind of wind and chill, but one with chillphobia from internal injury dreads even minor drafts. External contraction manifests in a stuffy nose which hampers breathing. Internal injury manifests itself in the mouth, hence the mouth cannot detect tastes, and there is abdominal disturbance. In external contraction evil *ch'i* is in excess, hence the patient speaks in a loud voice, beginning softly and then becoming louder. In internal injury, the patient's primordial *ch'i* is deficient, hence the patient speaks tiredly and timidly, the voice being heavy at first and then becoming lighter. Headache in external contraction occurs continuously, but headache in internal injury occurs intermittently. External contraction manifests fever on the back sides of the hands and no fever on the palms, whereas in internal injury fever occurs on the palms with no fever on the backs of the hands."

Li Tung-yuan (李東垣) said, "Pyrexia in feverish disease is the same as in external contraction." Hence, we cited the above information to aid clinical conformational identification.

3. *Tidal fever*

Tidal fever presents only thermophobia, no chillphobia. It occurs in the afternoon like the incoming tide, once every day at exactly the same time. The time falls within the *wei* (未) and *shen* (申) (1:00-5:00 PM) hours, corresponding to the sunlight yang earth that thrives in these hours. Evil that enters the stomach stagnates there and becomes a firm fever causing abdominal distention that resists pressing, constipation, spontaneous perspiration, and even delirium. The pulse is slippery, big, and forceful, or submerged and forceful. The condition requires purgation with *Ta-cheng-chi-tang* (大承氣湯 Major Rhubarb Combination). If the fever occurs three to five times dayly, it is ordinary pyrexia, not tidal fever.

Tidal fever is classified as firm or weak. The firm conformational tidal fever is as mentioned above, where the fever lingers throughout the day, culminating in the *wei* and *shen* hours. On the other hand, weak conformational tidal fever is such that in the morning there is no fever, the fever comes on in the afternoon or night, or the fever exhibits itself in the form of fever with internal annoyance, which is mostly due to chronic yin weakness disease. It is also observed in the late stage of feverish diseases. The treatment calls for *Ching-hao-pieh-chia-chien* (青蒿別甲煎 Ching-hao and Turtle Shell Combination).

4. *Alternating Chills and Fever*

Alternating chills and fever of feverish diseases resemble that of malaria, but differ in some respects. Malaria occurs every day or every other day at about the same time and lasts for a similar period of time. Alternating chills and fever, conversely, occur at different times, once to several times a day, and last for varying periods of time, with chillphobia being of shorter duration than fever. The evil of alternating chills and fever in the former is either located in the half-surface/half-interior area or lingers among the three warmers. If the evil is located in the half-surface/half-interior area, it is in the lesser yang meridian, and manifests the symptoms of thoracocostal distention and a chordal-slippery or chordal-quick pulse. It should be treated by clearing and dispersing the respiratory organs and harmonizing the condition with *Sang-chai-yin* (桑柴飲 Morus and Bupleurum Combination), or *Hsiao-chai-hu-tang-chia-chien* (小柴胡湯加減 Minor Bupleurum Combination modified). As for the evil that lingers among the three warmers, it does not cause costal distention, but exhibits in most cases a soft-quick or submerged-quick pulse due to moisture fever stagnating the *ch'i* domain and preventing the circulation of *ch'i,* as is frequently seen in moisture feverish disease.

Yeh Tien-shih (葉天士) said:

> The situation of evil lingering among the three warmers is just like that of the lesser yang stage of *shang han* diseases. The lesser yang disease is treated by harmonizing and resolving the surface and the interior. The former is treated by resolving the conditions of the upper and lower parts respectively, and varying the treatment in accordance with the conformation. An example is the recent use of apricot seed, magnolia bark, and hoelen, or the formula *Wen-tan-tang* (温膽湯 Bamboo and Hoelen Combination), which moves and purges. The reason for using such herbs is because the evil is still in the *ch'i* domain and we can expect to bring about shivering and sweating whereby the situation can be converted to a malarial condition, and treated as such.

To this statement Wang Mong-ying commented:

> By resolving the conditions of the upper and lower parts respectively, Yeh meant to open up the upper part with apricot seed, broaden the middle part with magnolia bark, and drain the lower part with hoelen. This treatment works on moist feverish disease or on those who used to have water stagnancy. Therefore, *Wen-tan-tang* (温膽湯) also can be used. If the condition is due to a wind feverish evil lingering in the *ch'i* domain, it requires cleansing the *ch'i.* This so-called "cleansing the *ch'i*" means to expand the *ch'i* in order to clear and lighten it. To this end, gardenia, scute, trichosanthes, and phragmites are used. As for the phrase "converted to a malarial condition",

it originally meant that as the ch'i circulates unobstructedly, the disease condition will change to malaria which, being an evil, can be guided and directed out of the body to effect a gradual healing of the disease."

Contemporary scholar Hsieh Li-heng made a rather clear and detailed explanation about this conversion to a malarial condition:

> When a feverish disease at its late stage turns again into alternating chills and fever like malaria, it is called "conversion to malaria". This occurs as a consequence of purgation and sweating treatments that have cleared and resolved the evils. The evils are then weakened but the normal *ch'i* has not yet recovered completely. The primordial *ch'i* then expels the residual evils from the interior toward the surface via the lesser yang area. Formerly, the yang evil was thriving alone and there was no chill. Now, yin fluid is gradually returning and being replenished, so chills and fever appear alternately. Formerly there was incessant scorching fever day and night. Now evils are retreating and normal *ch'i* is recovering; hence chills and fever occur and cease regularly.

5. *Spontaneous perspiration*

In feverish diseases, sweating that occurs spontaneously, not as a result of pyrexia, is called spontaneous perspiration. If fever remains unrelieved even though the patient has sweated, it should not be regarded as a surface weakness condition. It is called pathic sweating which is due to uncoordinated *jon* and *wei* (interior and surface) and presence of feverish fever on the surface to cause non-thorough sweating, and requires treatment with acrid, cool herbs to relieve the muscles and to bring forth orthodox sweating whereby the disease is healed. This is likened to the treatment of diarrhea accompanying fever with a *Cheng-chi-tang* (承氣湯 rhubarb-containing formulas) purgative. Such treatment employs the principle of "deobstruents for deobstruction".

Hsu Lin-tai (徐靈胎) said:

> Spontaneous perspiration is distinctly different from

hidrotic sweating. The former is due to uncoordinated *ying* (營) and *wei* (衛) (interior and surface regions), whereas the latter causes *ying* and *wei* to work in concert. The former injures the normal vitality while the latter dispels evils. If in the presence of spontaneous perspiration a sudorific is given to effect sweating, the *ying* and *wei* are coordinated, and spontaneous perspiration will then cease (Please see the *Shang han lei fang* 傷寒類方).

Lu Chiu-chih (陸九芝) of the Ching (清) dynasty said:

> A disease with the symptom of spontaneous perspiration is a hidrotic disease which should be treated by sweating to relieve the muscles. Sweating in the latter condition is a disease-ridding sweating and it is only this disease-ridding sweating that can arrest the sweating.

As evils enter the sunlight yang stage, symptoms such as profuse sweating, severe vexation and thirst, steaming pyrexia, and a surging and big pulse indicate a sunlight yang meridian conformation which should be treated by cleansing the fever with *Chu-yeh-shih-kao-tang* (竹葉石膏湯 Bamboo Leaf and Gypsum Combination). Vexation, thirst, and sweating will then cease automatically. In the event of a firm conformation of the sunlight yang viscus, there will certainly be constipation, fever, perspiration, coarse yellow tongue fur, and a quick and forceful pulse. This condition requires immediate purgation with *Cheng-chi-tang* (承氣湯 rhubarb-containing formulas) to quell the fever evil and effect cessation of sweating.

6. Night sweats

Sweating that occurs during sleep but ceases after waking is known as night sweats. It is a consequence of the *wei ch'i* (衛氣 protective vitality of the body surface) moving inward and circulating in the interior. The *wei ch'i* is thus unable to protect the surface and the evil fever then takes advantage of this unsolid surface condition, causing fluids to be discharged from the body. Hence, sweat comes out during sleep. On awakening and after sleep, the *wei ch'i* circulates on the surface again, hence sweating stops. In many conformations this is due to yin weakness and blood fever; in feverish diseases this is due to internal fever and an uncoordinated surface. *Ching-je-ku-piao-tang* (清熱固表湯 Gypsum and Lycium Bark Combination) is the principal formula to be used in both cases for cleansing the interior and harmonizing and coordinating the surface.

If after recovery from a feverish disease, the pulse is calm and the body exhibits a cool temperature, both urine and stool are clear and smooth, but spontaneous perspiration and night sweats continue incessantly, the condition can be treated as a weak conformation and *Huang-chi-ku-piao-tang* (黃耆固表湯 Astragalus and Wheat Combination) can be used as the preferred formula.

7. *Head sweats*

The head is the junction of all yangs. When evil fever is depressed and stagnated internally and finds no way to get out, it goes steaming up along the yang meridians toward the head, and fluids also are caused to ascend and converge at the head. As a consequence, the head sweats. This conformation is mostly due to a thriving fever of the sunlight yang meridian and manifests high fever, head sweats, constipation, and a quick and big pulse. It requires purgation with any of the three *Cheng-chi-tang* (承氣湯 rhubarb-containing formulas) to purge the fever and cause it to go downward so that the head sweats may cease. If there is no constipation, *Chu-yeh-shih-kao-tang* (竹葉石膏湯 Bamboo Leaf and Gypsum Combination) is used to cleanse and purge the stomachic fever.

8. *Limbic sweats*

Limbic sweats also belong to the sunlight yang meridian because the sunlight yang meridian is in charge of the stomach, and the stomach in turn is in charge of the four limbs. As fever gathers at the stomach, fluids overflow to the limbs. Hence, the limbs sweat. The condition requires purgation treatment.

9. *Sweating with tremors*

Sweating with tremors signifies a competition between the normal vitality and the evil that causes generalized trembling.

It portends that the evil is being weakened and normal vitality is recovering. At this moment we should keep calm instead of getting scared and disturbed, and wait for the sweating and tremors to continue. We should let the patient lie down quietly and comfortably, and have him take more hot water to aid the sweating so that the evil is sweated out and resolved. Before the tremors and sweating, the patient must experience quivering and limbic chills, a hidden pulse (a phenomenon of culminant yang resembling yin), and extreme obstruction becoming unblocked, a presymptom of sweating with tremors. The *Shang han lun* states, "A greater yang disease, not yet resolved, with interruption of pulse detected either superficially or deeply must undergo sweating with tremors before resolution of the disease." This passage indicates the same condition. If after the tremors and sweating, the pulse becomes calm and the body cool, and the patient feels a desire to eat, it is a sign that the evil has retreated and the normal vitality has recovered. Otherwise, the residual evil that remains uncleansed will cause a recurrence of the fever, and further sweating with tremors is necessary to bring about the resolution. Sweating with tremors is more commonly seen in feverish diseases, and scarcely seen in afflications from an external contraction of winds and chills. When a person who used to have a weak constitution suffers from a feverish disease and the normal vitality is weak while the feverish evil is thriving, sweating with tremors will occur as the evil fever invades and competes with the normal vitality in the interior. If it turns out that the normal vitality prevails over the evil, then the patient trembles and sweats and the disease heals. If the patient only trembles without perspiration, it indicates the normal vitality has not yet gotten the upper hand and thus cannot drive out the evil. At this moment we may augment the normal vitality to dispel the evil, or add to the herbal formulas some yin-nourishing components to nourish the source of sweat so that the sweat can come out and the condition can be resolved. As mentioned earlier, in the presence of a tremor it is necessary to drink more hot water to augment sweating. It also means we need to supply fluids to nourish the source of sweat. Fang Yu (方隅) of the Ming (明) dynasty said in his *I lin sheng mo* (醫林繩墨), "During trembling, drugs should not be given. They do not help, but only cause disaster. To promote sweating, just drink more ginger decoction." However, since the ginger decoction is hot-natured and hence unsuitable for feverish diseases, it is better to drink hot water.

10. Headache

Headache in feverish diseases is due to a thriving feverish evil that flushes up to the head and eyes and differs from the headache in common wind and chill afflictions. Wind- and chill-caused headaches can be resolved by dispersing the surface. Whereas the headache in feverish diseases cannot be treated simply by surface dispersion methods, if it occurs at the initial stage and the pain occurs at the back and top of the head, the tongue fur is thin and white, there is fever, and a slippery and quick pulse can be detected. Although these symptoms belong to a surface conformation and are similar to the symptoms of a greater yang headache, the treatment requires simultaneously cleansing the interior and resolving the surface with formulas such as *Sang-chu-yin* (桑菊飲 Morus and Chrysanthemum Combination) and herbs like raw gypsum, vitex, and camellia. If the patient has swelling pain at the forehead, or aching of the eyebrow bones, earache, fever, annoying thirst, and a slippery-quick pulse, these belong to an internal conformation, like a sunlight yang headache. The condition requires cleansing of the surface and interior with formulas like *Pai-hu-tang* (白虎湯 Gypsum Combination), *Sheng-chiang-san* (升降散 Silkworm and Rhubarb Formula), and *Shuang-chieh-san* (雙解散 Siler and Mentha Formula). If the aching appears at the two upper corners of the forehead, or there are alternating chills and fever signifying a semi-surface/semi-interior condition, it is a lesser yang headache, and requires treatment with *Tseng-shun-ta-chai-hu-tang* (增損大柴胡湯 Major Bupleurum Combination modified) together with vitex, or camellia. The foregoing types of headache are due to diseases of the three yang meridians, and require treatment by cleansing and purging the internal fever. Once the internal *ch'i* is unblocked, headaches cease spontaneously. In summer feverish disease the headache is more violent. If the symptoms of headache, vomiting, and high fever are not controlled, they will promptly turn into coma. This kind of headache cannot be controlled by ordinary drugs. It requires *Hsi-chiao-fen* (犀角粉 Rhinoceros Horn Powder), *Ling-yang-chiao-fen* (羚羊角粉 Antelope Horn Powder), *Chu-fang-chih-pao-tan* (局方至寶丹 Rhinoceros and Succinum Formula) or even *Huei-su-san* (回蘇散 Rhinoceros and Cinnabar Formula) which is especially efficacious.

Diseases of the greater and lesser yin meridians exhibit generalized fever but no headache. Absolute yin disease has headache but no generalized fever, dry heaves, vomiting, drivel, and cold arms and legs. It required *Wu-chu-yu-tang* (吳茱萸湯 Evodia Combination). Feverish diseases never manifest absolute yin headaches because headaches in feverish diseases must be accompanied by generalized fever, although there may also be vomiting. This is different from the absolute yin headache of *shang han* diseases; that is, the absolute yin headache has no generalized fever, whereas a headache in feverish diseases does.

11. Vertigo

Vertigo refers to a dizzy and whirling sensation in the head, with a blackening of vision. It is differentiated according to whether the condition is new, chronic, weak, or firm. Sudden onset of vertigo belongs to a firm condition due to an up-flushing of liver fire. Sometimes, fever scorches and turns fluids into sputum; the sputum fever then wells up causing vertigo, expectoration of sputum, slobbering, and a slippery-quick or chordal-quick pulse. At the beginning of a feverish disease, vertigo is often a firm symptom, and requires treatment by cleansing the liver and extinguishing winds. The formulas indicated are *Ling-yang-kou-teng-tang-chia-chien* (羚羊鈎藤湯加減 Antelope Horn and Gambir Combination modified); or this formula with pinellia, citrus, and bamboo added. In the latter stage of feverish diseases, vertigo is mostly a sign of yin-weakness which requires treatment by filling up the yin and submerging the yang, using formulas such as *Yu-nu-chien* (玉女煎 Rehmannia and Gypsum Combination) with fresh venus shells, *ho-sho-wu,* and chrysanthemum; *Liu-wei-ti-huang-wan* (六味地黃丸 Rehmannia Six Formula), or *Sang-ma-wan* (桑麻丸 Morus and Linum Formula).

12. Generalized aching, heaviness, and peripheral soreness

The symptoms of generalized aching, arthralgia, chillphobia, anhidrosis, and a floating-tense pulse are due to a *shang han* disease, and require acrid and warm herbs to produce sweating. Feverish diseases also exhibit generalized aching, headache, and fever. They resemble *shang han* diseases, but have a slippery-quick pulse, dry nose, and thirst as the distinctive symptoms. The cause of these symptoms is fever obstructed in the triple warmers and the resultant blockage between the surface and the interior. Treatment requires fever-cleansing and detoxifying to unblock and purge the feverish evil, using formulas such as *Sheng-chiang-san* (升降散 Silkworm and Rhubarb Formula), and *Tseng-shun-shuang-chieh-san* (增損雙解散 Siler and Mentha Formula modified). Moist feverish disease also exhibits generalized aching though its chief symptom is generalized heaviness; additionally it manifests a filthy, greasy face, scant red urine, and a depressed, quick and inactive pulse. Treatment employs fragrant herbs to resolve turbidity. A formula for these conditions is *Huo-pu-hsia-ling-tang* (藿朴夏苓湯 Agastache and Polyporus Combination). If the surface evils have been resolved and the fever is gone but soreness still persists throughout the body, it is because the evil has not been completely cleansed and has flowed into various meridians. This condition calls for *Shu-lo-chu-feng-tang* (舒絡祛風湯 Lonicera Stem and Clematis Combination). Chou Yang-chun (周揚俊) of the Ching (清) dynasty said, "Generalized soreness is treated by dispersing the surface as the chief method."

13. Bowel movements

Constipation, sticky and mucilaginous stool, watery diarrhea, and feverish diarrhea are the four most commonly seen symptoms in feverish diseases. They are conformations of feverish evil in the interior.

Constipation indicates the presence of a fever evil in the interior of the body. While the normal *ch'i* is thriving, evils enter the sunlight yang meridian, causing internally obstructed and stagnated fever, internally bound night soil, and gradual formation of hard stool. In this case the tongue fur must be yellow and thick, the patient has incessant tidal fever, and a quick and forceful pulse. Treatment calls for purgation to unblock bowel movement and discharge the hardened stool, thereby spontaneously resolving the stagnant fever.

Sticky and mucilaginous stool is due to feverish fever bound internally where the stool is not hard, but has been steamed by the fever to become sticky, mucilaginous, and malodorous. If bowel movement occurs spontaneously without the use of a purgative, the toxic fever is thus provided with a descendant path. We should then employ a "deobstruent for loose bowels" to aid the toxin-expelling effect in order that the fever may recede and the conformation ameliorate after the dirty, turbid, and sticky substance has been completely cleansed. The text under the formula for a *shang han* disease with internal firmness states that in the presence of an overwhelming fever in a feverish disease, purge it at once. Internal firmness is a condition of obstruction, distention, aridity, denseness, and solidity. An overwhelming fever (that should be purged at once) indicates a condition that can be purged only in the presence of yellow tongue fur and cardioabdominal obstruction and distention, without having all symptoms of a purgeable conformation appearing at the same time. *Ta-cheng-chi-tang* (大承氣湯 Major Rhubarb Combination) was originally formulated for dispelling toxicity, not specifically for treating constipation. If on observation of sticky and mucilaginous stool, the physician erroneously prescribes a tonic and astringent formula, it will cause erosion and rotting of the stomach and intestine, leading to disastrous consequences.

Watery diarrhea is a condition of feverish evil located in the interior, whereby the stool hardens and cannot descend and stinking water then flows between the stool and the intestinal wall. The patient must have generalized fever, annoying thirst and a slippery and quick pulse. Treatment makes use of a "deobstruent for loose bowels" and purgatives are used to discharge hard stool. The diarrhea will then cease spontaneously. If the physician mistakes the condition for diarrhea due to splenic weakness and prescribes a tonic and astringent herb, the constipation will become more obstinate, and the diarrhea more serious; much harm can ensue.

Feverish diarrhea manifests yellowish-red stool, a drastic downpouring of stool, a burning sensation at the anus on defecation, annoying thirst, dry mouth, harshness in urination, and a quick, rushing or surging, big pulse. Treatment calls for *Ko-ken-huang-lien-huang-chin-tang* (葛根黃連黃芩湯 Pueraria, Coptis, and Scute Combination) with lonicera, and *I-yuan-san* (益元散 Talc and Cinnabar Formula).

If no bowel movement occurs after recovery from a feverish disease, it is due to a fluid insufficiency for which the patient should not be purged needlessly. After the patient gradually gains his appetite, fluids then circulate to moisten the colon spontaneously. Alternatively, *Tseng-yeh-tang* (增液湯 Rehmannia, Ophiopogon, and Scrophularia Combination) can be used for moistening purposes.

Stools of yellow-brown color are normal; purely brown indicates fever; a dark brown color indicates a more severe fever; and a black color, the severest fever.

14. Urine

By observing the urine color we can tell the intensity of an internal fever. When a fever evil enters the interior, the urine color is yellow. As the fever becomes strong, the urine color becomes red. If the color is dark red with a black tint, the fever has entered the blood domain. These conditions all require *Liu-i-san* (六一散 Talc and Licorice Formula) with anemarrhena, phellodendron, gardenia, and bamboo leaves to cleanse the urinary bladder.

Frequent, short, and harsh urination with pain is evidence of fever bound in the urinary bladder, which should be treated by cleansing the lower warmer with *Pa-cheng-san* (八正散 Dianthus Formula). Oliguria in feverish diseases indicates fever entering the urinary bladder. It calls for treatment with *Szu-ling-san* (四苓散 Hoelen Four Herb Formula), *Chu-ling-tang* (豬苓湯 Polyporus Combination), or *Liu-i-san* (六一散 Talc and Licorice Formula). If there is also constipation, the bowel must first be moved. Once the bowel moves, urine flows spontaneously. Oliguria with thirst is a sign of fever in the upper warmer, which requires bland-tasting herbs to seep out water. The formula called for is *Wu-*

ling-san (五苓散 Hoelen Five Herb Formula). Oliguria without thirst indicates fever in the lower warmer and should be treated with bitter, chilly herbs together with acrid, warm herbs to cause the water to evaporate. The formula indicated is *Tzu-shen-tung-kuan-wan* (滋腎通關丸 Phellodendron, Anemarrhena, and Cinnamon Formula).

As for obstructed urine (urinary retention), it is due to a stagnated and obstructed fever evil and an impaired, evaporating function of the urinary bladder.

Chang Shih-wan (張石頑) said in his *Shang han hsu lun* (傷寒緒論 An Introduction to the *Shang han lun*):

> As evil *ch'i* accumulates in the lower warmer it binds there undispersed. Then the lower abdomen becomes distended and painful because urine is blocked. If excessive water is taken, it is stagnated and retained, or the lower warmer will have excess fever. The stomach can become distended and jaundice will occur.

For these conditions, diuresis is the proper treatment. Formulas such as *Wu-ling-san* (五苓散 Hoelen Five Herb Formula), *Pa-cheng-san* (八正散 Dianthus Formula), and *Tzu-shen-wan* (滋腎丸 Phellodendron, Anemarrhena, and Cinnamon Formula) may be used after appropriate modifications to suit the respective conditions, or with the addition of a little asarum to unblock the urinary obstruction. The white parts of scallions that are fried hot and placed as a fomentation on the navel are also effective. If a little musk is applied before the scallions, the results will be even better.

15. Scrotal contraction

Scrotal contraction appearing in feverish diseases is due to sunlight yang fever sinking into the absolute yin meridian. Because the absolute yin meridian encircles the genitals, when the absolute yin meridian is scorched by fever, muscles contract and undergo spasms. The condition expresses itself in the form of scrotal contraction in men and nipple contraction in women. Treatment calls for liver cleansing and fever purgation. Once the fever is cleansed, scrota relax spontaneously. If the condition is accompanied by constipation, distention and hardening pain of the lower abdomen, thirst, annoying distention, red and scant urine, and a forceful pulse, it should be purged at once with *Ta-cheng-chi-tang* (大承氣湯 Major Rhubarb Combination). The *Chung tsang ching* (中藏經) says, "Scrotal contraction and lingual curling are lethal symptoms." Feverish diseases that develop to such a stage as to exhibit lingual curling and scrotal contraction are really dangerous. Because when evil fever scorches internally, manifesting a dry tongue without saliva and an arid mouth and lips, it is necessary to purge immediately in order to preserve the yin so that the patient may possibly be saved.

This conformation belongs to a lesser yin weakness chill with which the patient must have a submerged and minute pulse, limbic chilling, a dark face, and asthma, or spontaneous perspiration of cold sweat. It should be treated by urgently restoring yang with *Szu-ni-tang* (四逆湯 Aconite and G.L. Combination) with ginseng. However, since feverish diseases have no yin conformation, mistaking the conformation for a chill and treating it as such will lead to danger and death.

16. Bitter, sweet, and arid mouth

A bitter, sweet or arid mouth is a manifestation of a fever conformation. These qualities are exhibited not only in feverish diseases, but also in external contractions of winds and chills where there is internal fever. A bitter mouth is due to arid fever, and requires *Yu-nu-chien* (玉女煎 Rehmannia and Gypsum Combination), *Tseng-shun-san-huang-shih-kao-tang* (增損三黄石膏湯 Gypsum, Coptis, and Scute Combination modified), or *Pai-hu-tang* (白虎湯 Gypsum Combination). A sweet mouth is due to moist fever and requires *Hsieh-huang-san* (瀉黄散 Siler and Licorice Formula), or *Wen-tan-tang* (温膽湯 Bamboo and Hoelen Combination) together with anemarrhena, phellodendron, and eupatorium. An arid mouth is present either in the beginning or the late stage of a disease. If an arid mouth is observed at the beginning, it is due to a firm fever and should be treated with *Chu-yeh-shih-kao-tang* (竹葉石膏湯 Bamboo Leaf and Gypsum Combination) and *Yu-nu-chieh* (玉女煎 Rehmannia and Gypsum Combination). Arid mouth occurring in the late stage of a disease is due to a weakness fever and fluid deficiently, and requires nourishing the stomach *yang* with *Wu-chih-yin* (五汁飲 Pear

Five Juice Combination), or *I-kuan-chien* (一貫煎 Glehnia and Rehmannia Combination) with scrophularia and schizandra. Tai Pei-shan (戴北山) said, "A bitter mouth is evidence of a fever conformation, a symptom which helps us decide whether it is a chill or fever conformation."

17. Thirst

Presence or absence of thirst tells whether the evil resides in the interior of the body or on the surface. When winds and chills occur on the surface, there is no thirst. Only after these evils have entered the interior and turned into fever does thirst begin to appear. However, in feverish diseases thirst occurs right from the onset. As the *Shang han lun* (傷寒論) states, "A greater yang disease with fever and thirst but without chillphobia is a feverish disease." As for moist feverish disease, it occurs before the moisture has turned into aridity; the patient feels thirsty but has no desire to drink. After the moisture is transformed into aridity, the patient then is thirsty and desires to drink water. A patient with a feverish disease favors cool drinks; with moisture feverish disease, hot drinks. The intensity of thirst tells the severity of the fever: mild thirst indicates a mild fever, and strong thirst, a strong fever. In general, feverish or fever diseases with severe thirst, causing the patient to drink large quantities of water, have fever in the *ch'i* domain or fever bound in the sunlight yang area. If fever is in the *ch'i* domain, the symptoms are generalized fever, spontaneous perspiration, yellow tongue fur, and a surging and big pulse. The condition calls for treatment with *Pai-hu-tang* (白虎湯 Gypsum Combination), *Tseng-shun-san-huang-shih-kao-tang* (增損三黃石膏湯), or *Chu-yeh-shih-kao-tang* (竹葉石膏湯 Bamboo Leaf and Gypsum Combination). If the fever is bound in the sunlight yang area, there is also generalized fever, spontaneous perspiration, yellow thick tongue fur, abdominal distention resisting pressing, dry hardened stool, and a slippery-big or submerged-forceful pulse. It requires *San-cheng-chi-tang* (三承氣湯 either of the three rhubarb-containing purgatives) or *Pai-hu-cheng-chi-tang* (白虎承氣湯) to cleanse, resolve, and purge the fever; thirst will be spontaneously resolved then. If fever is in the blood domain instead of the *ch'i* domain, and if there is thirst, it does not cause excessive drinking. The treatment calls for *Ching-ying-tang* (清營湯 Rhinoceros and Scrophularia Combination) or a similar formula. If thirst occurs in the late stage of feverish diseases, when the yin fluids have been injured and arid thirst is exhibited, *I-wei-tang* (益胃湯 Glehnia and Ophiopogon Combination), *I-kuang-chien* (一貫煎), *Tseng-yeh-tang* (增液湯 Rehmannia, Ophiopogon, and Scrophularia Combination), or *Wu-chih-yin* (五汁飲 Pear Five Juice Combination) can be chosen.

D) Pulse palpation

1. The theory that pulses are essentially ch'i

When the ancients referred to "diagnosis by palpation" they meant specifically diagnosis by pulse palpation. The *Nan ching* (Classic of Medical Difficulties) states under the first difficulty:

> Each of the twelve meridians has moving pulses. But why do we take pulses at the *chun* site to determine the lively, deadly, favorable and critical states of the viscera? Because the *chun* site is a place where all pulses meet and it reflects the pulsation of the hand-greater yin meridian.

The lungs receive all pulses and are regarded as forming an umbrella for the viscera. The *ch'is* from the viscera all come steaming up to the lungs, with changes in the *ch'is* being reflected at the *chun* site. The reason we can diagnose the pulses of the various viscera at the *chun* site is because the visceral *ch'is* go along with the pulmonary *ch'i* and appear at the *tai yuan* point (about the *chun* site), not because all visceral pulses collect at this site. From this we can see that the pulsations are caused by the flowing of *ch'is.* Hence, Chuei Chia-yen (崔嘉言) said, "Pulses do not move by themselves. They come along with *ch'i.*" Tao Chiu-cheng (陶九成) of the Yuan (元) dynasty said in his *Chuo keng lu* (輟耕錄 Interrupted Farming), "Pulses are of blood. Pulses do not move by themselves. *Ch'i* moves them." Therefore, the essential purpose of pulse diagnosis is to determine the condition of the *ch'i.* It has been said, "With gastric *ch'i* one lives; without gastric *ch'i* one dies."

The *Chung tsang ching* (中藏經) states:

> Pulses precede *ch'i* and blood. If *ch'i* and blood are exuberant, pulses are exuberant; if *ch'i* and blood deteriorate, pulses will deteriorate. If *ch'i* and blood have fever, the pulses become quickened. If *ch'i* and blood are cold, the pulses are slowed down. If *ch'i* and blood are minute, the pulses are weak. If *ch'i* and blood are normal, the pulses are moderate.

Hence, whenever a pulse is referred to, the corresponding *ch'i* and blood are also mentioned and the *ch'i* is especially emphasized. However, since *ch'i* is intangible, shapeless, and colorless, we can only detect it in a moderate pulse. Being moderate means mild, gentle and calm, but not slow. It is neither rushing nor slow, but gentle, tender, and mild. No matter if it is a sick or normal pulse, if the pulse exhibits a gentle, tender, and mild character, it is considered an indication of gastric *ch'i.* The *Yu chi chen tsang lun* chapter (玉機眞藏論 An Expounding On Authentic Viscera Preserved in a Jade Desk) in the *Nei ching* (內經) states, "A pulse with a weak and slippery character is with gastric *ch'i.*" Chang Ching-yueh (張景岳) said, "It is important for a pulse to have 'spirit'". Here, "spirit" means "gastric *ch'i*".

Ancients said:

> Sphygmology is occult and difficult to understand. What I get in my mind cannot be spoken. What can be written in words and described verbally are only signs and facts. As for the divine metaphysical aspect of sphygmology, it can only be mentally apprehended; otherwise, we will not be able to totally understand the minute details of its profound knowledge.

Therefore, in studying sphygmology, if we only learn about the tangible evidence of pulsations and ignore the traceless spirit and *ch'i*, we are a great distance astray from the correct way.

One may say the *chun* site is just a small area no larger than one cubic inch, and imagine the pulse will be the same all along a given blood vessel, but this is not true. Is it not too miraculous and metaphysical to say that one can distinguish pulses corresponding to the five solid and six hollow viscera and can tell whether the outcome will be favorable or disastrous or whether the patient will live or die?

It should be noted here that this effect is due to the action of *ch'is* which manifests different sphygmological conditions within the same blood vessel. This can be likened to playing the flute: different holes along the flute generate different tones. The principle behind the way the flute produces different tones at different locations is similar to that of vascular pulses. Hence without blowing, the flute does not sound, and without the action of the *ch'i,* the pulses do not move either. From the movement of air, the flute gives forth five tones and six pitches and the blood vessel generates different pulses corresponding to the five solid and six hollow viscera.

2. Pulses are distinguished as being true, false, empty, and forceful.

Diseases are distinguished by their conformations as being chill, fever, empty, or forceful, though they should be considered with pulse palpation before an accurate diagnosis can be made. However, pulses are also differentiated into true, false, empty, and forceful. The identity of an empty or forceful pulse lies in a submerged pulse. For example, on light pressing the pulse feels surging and big, suggesting a firm conformation. However, on heavy pressing, it disappears or becomes thin, weak and forceless. The condition should be regarded and treated as a weakness conformation. If the pulse is unpalpable on light or medium pressing, but on heavy pressing it feels slippery, coarse, and forceful, the condition should be treated as a firm fever conformation.

Also, some people used to have pulses belonging to the six yin meridians, those pulses being finer than normal. This condition should not be taken as a weakness conformation. Some other people used to have pulses belonging to the six yang meridians, the pulses being bigger than normal. The condition should not be taken as a firm conformation. The preceding conditions are physiological phenomena and the pulses so expressed should not be taken as being pathogenic. We must first know about the usual conditions, then we can understand the varied and altered conditions. If someone has no pulse in his hands, but he is strong and without any ailment, we cannot take this as a case of that person having a death pulse.

Sometimes the pulse agrees with the conformation and sometimes not. For example, in feverish diseases, a surging, big, slippery, and quick pulse matches the conformation. Nevertheless, if the pulse is submerged, thin, and minute, the pulse and conformation do not agree with each other. Chang Chung-ching (張仲景) of the Han (漢) dynasty said, "A yin disease with a yang pulse allows survival, a yang disease with a yin pulse leads to death." Besides, some patients do not exhibit a death pulse even when they are in a critical state and going to die. This is often found in the senile. Therefore, we have to refer jointly to the other information obtained from diagnoses by observation, olfaction, auscultation, and inquiry.

The *Nei ching* also states, "Solitary 'big' portends illness; solitary 'fine' portends illness." For example, among the pulses of the six parts, the pulse of one part alone might manifest a slippery, big, and forceful character while the other parts are submerged, fine, and forceless. We must pay special attention to this solitary big pulse, and consider it a firm condition. Contrarily, if the pulse of one of the six parts exhibits a minute, weak, and forceless character, while the other parts' pulses are slippery and big, we must pay attention to the solitary fine pulse and consider it as reflecting a weak condition. This is expressed by the maxim, "Dishonesty lies in solitariness."

Hsu Ling-tai (徐靈胎) said:

> Symptom and pulse may differ from each other. Sometimes, the symptom is considered the true indicator, and sometimes the pulse is considered the true indicator. When the symptom is to be followed, death is predicted in the presence of a critical condition despite an extremely fluent pulse palpation. When the pulse is to be followed, survival is predicted in the presence of a normal pulse despite the manifestation of an extremely dangerous symptom.

Hence, in clinical identification of conformations, whether one is to follow the symptom and disregard the pulse or vice versa, close attention and careful understanding are necessary for an accurate synthesis of the diagnostic information in order to avoid iatrogenic errors.

3. *Frequently observed pulses in feverish diseases*

The following are pulses frequently observed in feverish diseases. However, since pulses do not represent fixed types of diseases, the twenty-eight types of pulses must be kept in mind and combined with symptoms before a final diagnosis can be made.

The *Lun chi chen chih pien* (論疾診尺篇 Chapter on Diagnosing the *Chih* Site for the Consultation of Diseases) in the *Ling su* (靈樞) volume of the *Nei ching* (内經) states, "When the skin over the *chih* site is excessively hot, and the pulse is thriving and irritable, it is a feverish disease." The so-called thriving and irritable pulse denotes surging, long, slippery, and quick characteristics. The *Ping jen chi hsiang lun* (平人氣象論 Expounding on a Normal Individual's *Ch'i* Condition) in the *Su wen* (素問) volume of the *Nei ching* (内經) states, "When there are three pulse beats during one inhalation, and three beats during one exhalation, the pulse is agitated in character, signalling fever on the *chih* site, it is a feverish disease." This is the same condition as the preceding passage that mentioned feverish *chih* skin and a thriving and agitated pulse.

Chou Yu-tsai (周禹載) of the Ching (清) dynasty said in his *Shu i chuan shu* (暑疫全書 A Complete Work on Summer Plague):

> The pulses of feverish diseases are mostly located in muscles. The pulses are not very buoyant, and pulses on the right wrist are more thriving than those on the left wrist. They are actually due to fever stagnated in the interior. If pulses on the left hand are thriving or floating, it must be due to a severe contraction of winds and chills.

Sometimes a stagnant fever evil gives rise to a submerged, hidden pulse that tends to exhaust. However, on such occasions, the pulse must feel forceful when we press our fingers deeply to the bone. This is a phenomenon known as "the deeper the fever, the deeper the chilling." When the fire evil is suppressed and stagnated, both *ch'i* and blood are blocked and stagnated. It requires purgation and a toxin-expelling method to unblock *ch'i* and blood, thereby restoring the pulse.

In the beginning of feverish diseases, when there is fever (but no chillphobia), dry mouth and throat, thirst, and a surging and quick pulse in most cases (or even submerged and hidden pulse), treatment with acrid, warm herbs to cause sweating is prohibited.

In feverish diseases with fever in the interior and on the surface, a submerged and hidden pulse that is neither surging nor quick but forceful underneath the fingers, the condition should not be mistaken for weak chill. Hence, *shang han* diseases are judged mostly by pulse, whereas feverish diseases are judged mostly by conformation.

Feverish diseases exhibiting surging, long, slippery, or quick pulses are mild; those exhibiting submerged and hidden pulses are grave; while those exhibiting obstructed and interrupted pulses are the worst and known as pulse faint. In contrast to this, limbic chilling or even generalized coldness is known as body faint, which is termed by Chang Chung-ching (張仲景) "yang faint" and is characterized by the principle that the deeper (stronger) the chill, the deeper (stronger) the fever, or if the chill is mild, the fever is also mild. It is mandatory that the condition be purged and exterminated as late as possible. Please also refer to the article "Yang conformation resembling yin conformation."

4. Identification of death pulses and conformations

(a) The *Ping je lun* (評熱論 Chapter Commenting on Fever) in the *Su wen* (素問) states: "In some feverish diseases in which fever often returns after cessation of perspiration, the pulse is agitated and rushing and cannot be reduced by sweating; the patient has delirium, unintelligible speech, and an inability to eat. The disease is known as interchange of yin and yang. Here "interchange" means death. On this, Yu Chou-wu (尤拙吾) commented, "Interchange does not mean intercourse but a disorderly derangement."

(b) The *Yu pan pien* (玉版篇 The Jade Press Chapter) in the *Su wen* (素問) states, "Feverish diseases with extreme weakness lead to death." Wu Chu-tung (吳鞠通) said, "Patients with feverish diseases have extremely weakened essence and blood, and thus have no yin to overcome the feverish fever, hence death."

(c) The *Je ping pien* (熱病篇 Chapter on Fever Diseases) in the *Ling shu* (靈樞) states, "Excessive body fever with a calm pulse palpated superficially or deeply should not be treated with acupuncture. Acupuncture is prohibited because the symptom is lethal." That is, a yin pulse in the presence of a yang conformation indicates the normal vitality cannot overcome the evil, hence death.

(d) The *Je ping pien* (熱病篇 Chapter on Fever Diseases) in the *Ling shu* (靈樞) states, "A patient suffering from a fever disease for seven to eight days with a minute and fine pulse, hematuria, and dry mouth will die in one and a half days; if the pulse is intermittent, he will die in one day.

Wu Chu-tung (吳鞠通) commented:

> The evil *ch'i* has entered deeply into the lower warmer, forcing blood out through the urine, hence causing hematuria. The renal essence is exhausted, and there is no yin fluid to flow upward, hence there is a dry mouth. A minute and fine pulse indicates exhaustion not only in yin essence, but also in yang *ch'i,* which is a prominent lethal symptom. If the pulse is forceful, the disease can be healed.

(e) The same chapter above also states, "In a fever disease that has been perspired, if the pulse remains agitated and thriving, it is a culminant state of a yin pulse and portends death; if after perspiration the pulse become calm, the disease is healable." Wu Chu-tang (吳鞠通) said, "An agitated and thriving pulse appearing after perspiration is a culminant yin-weakness state. Hence, death. However, if the condition is appropriately treated with sweet and cool drugs, the patient sometimes can survive."

(f) The chapter above also states, "In a fever disease if there is no perspiration but the pulse remains agitated and thriving, it is the culminant state of a yang pulse; if the agitated and thriving pulse becomes calm after perspiration, the patient may survive." Wu Chu-tang (吳鞠通) said, "As yang thrives and reaches its culminant state, yin will have no place to stay: hence death."

(g) The above chapter also states, "There are nine conditions of fever diseases to which acupuncture should not be applied. These conditions are lethal: 1. Anhidrosis, ruddy cheeks, and retching; 2. Diarrhea with an excessively distended abdomen; 3. Blurred vision with incessant fever; 4. Fever with abdominal distention in infants and the old; 5. Anhidrosis, vomiting, and discharge of blood; 6. Erosion of the tongue texture with incessant fever; 7. Cough accompanied by epistaxis, together with anhidrosis, or perspiration which does not occur to the lower limbs; 8. Marrow fever; 9. Fever together with convulsions, lumbar bending, muscular spasms and flaccidity, lockjaw, and gnashing of teeth. Acupuncture used with these nine conditions is prohibited because of the lethal symptoms.

Wu Chu-tung (吳鞠通) said:

> Acupuncture is prohibited, but sometimes sufferers may be healed with herbal drugs. Acupuncture can purge and unblock, and is fastest at unblocking obstructed fever. As for replenishing the yin to preserve the fluids, acupuncture has its shortcomings; herbal decoctions are good at this.

The abovementioned conditions are listed as incurable symptoms in the *Nei ching* (內經), but are mostly curable nowadays through the joint application of Western and Chinese herbal medicine.

Hua Tuo (華佗) said in his *Chung tsang ching* (中藏經):

> A feverish disease lasting for three or four days without perspiration but with a big and rushing pulse is lethal. A feverish disease with a thin and minute pulse that moves to and fro unsmoothly and an obstruction in the chest signal death. A feverish disease without perspiration, or with perspiration that does not occur to the lower limbs also portends death.
>
> A feverish disease lasting for seven to eight days in which perspiration should occur but does not together with an interruption of pulse is lethal.
>
> A feverish disease lasting for seven to eight days

with anhidrosis, agitation, and madness, parched black mouth and tongue, and a pulse that is nevertheless thin and weak is lethal.

A feverish disease without perspiration but with an excessively thriving pulse indicates death.

A feverish disease with perspiration but an uncalm pulse that moves to and fro, becoming big, means death.

All of these lethal diseases cited by Hua Tuo (華佗) are due to exhaustion in the yin *ch'i,* a symptom of thriving evil against weakened primordial *ch'i.*

Epilogue

Following the translation of *Shang han lun* and *Chin kuei yao lueh* – both originally written by Chang Chung-ching, the medical sage of China – we now present to our readers this translation of Wu Chu-tung's *Wen ping tiao pien* (Detailed Analysis of Feverish Diseases). The three books together constitute a trilogy on Chinese herbal medicine.

In order to supplement Chang's works, Wu Chu-tung endeavored to write a book dealing solely with feverish diseases. Mimicking the writing style of *Shang han lun* and *Chin kuei yao lueh,* Wu described feverish diseases in articles and systematically grouped them into three volumes according to the three warmers of the body (that is, by the particular warmer that a disease attacks). To each article he added commentary to further illuminate the meaning. In so doing he wanted there to be no guessing or misunderstanding as happened with *Shang han lun* and *Chin kuei yao lueh* due to lack of annotations to the articles.

As one can see from this book by Wu Chu-tung, feverish diseases are mostly treated with cool or cold herbs together with some acrid, moistening or diuretic herbs. In Chang's eyes, feverish diseases can be included in one or more stages of *shang han* diseases, depending on the symptoms manifested. Chang was aware that a *shang han* disease does not necessarily begin at the greater yang stage and then move inward; it may begin in any of the six stages. If it begins in the hand-greater yin stage, it may develop into a feverish disease and all symptoms may be treated accordingly. Hence, feverish disease is just a part of *shang han* disease. Medical books like *Shang han lun* and *Chin kuei yao lueh* that give principles, rules of treatment, and brief statements could not include all diseases encountered throughout history, nor could they provide detailed descriptions, especially in a time when paper was scarce and printing techniques were still primitive. Books were made of bamboo or wood strips, on which the words of the text were painstakingly inscribed, and so we cannot expect Chang Chung-ching to have provided more detail despite the great help it may have rendered toward the understanding of his doctrine. To Chang's surprise, subsequent people (a few geniuses excepted) could not learn much about feverish diseases from the statements scattered throughout his book. Therefore, Wu Chu-tung with his outstanding talent wrote this book to expand upon Chang Chung-ching's work on feverish diseases. Wu not only developed the concept of feverish disease to a fuller extent, but also provided a detailed exposition of Chang's theory, upon which he drew liberally in his own articles. Actually, Wu's theory is based on Chang's; Wu just did the exposition work for Chang, and developed "feverish disease" into a discrete branch. Therefore, reading Wu's work will help one understand Chang's work better, and that is why we recommend the reader read Chang's books vertically and Wu's horizontally.

Also, in order to avoid missing any bit of knowledge concerning the identification, discrimination, and treatment of feverish diseases or problems related thereto, Wu added many independent monographs to the end of the three main volumes. Because Wu firmly attributed the etiology of feverish diseases to meteorological factors or other of Mother Nature's influences, he began this book with the "Etiology of Disease" chapter in which he cited many passages from *Nei ching* to serve as theoretical bases for his writing. However, the reader might not understand the concept of Chinese cosmology, and so the author added to this chapter a brief statement about the celestial phases and terrestrial terms, introducing the theory and calculation rules of phaseotermology. "Phaseotermology" is one of the many terms we have devised for the English version of this book, because in Chinese culture, especially in Chinese herbal medicine, there are many concepts and terms not having English counterparts. Therefore, we have to create terms in order to render a clear description. It is generally believed that this aspect of Chinese culture is among the most difficult to translate, because it is conceptual and has no Western equivalent.

After reading this book, we can see that the author tried earnestly to expound and clarify for his readers the subtle aspects of Chinese herbal medicine as it relates to feverish diseases. His efforts and contributions are as glorious and great as his knowledge and experience of feverish diseases, and for this he deserves our respect.

My hearty thanks are due to Dr. Hong-yen Hsu for his great contributions to present-day Chinese herbal medicine. Without his beneficence in introducing and promoting Chinese herbal medicine in the West, our readers would not be able to read this translation at this time. It is our wish that the publication of this book contribute to the healing arts and help human beings enjoy a brighter and healthier tomorrow.

Wang Su-yen
Brion Research Institute of Taiwan
December 1984

Bibliography

1. Chao, S. C., Hu, D. B., and Liou, C. Y., *The Breadth and Width of Feverish Diseases* (Wen ping tsung heng, 溫病縱橫). Szechuan: People's Health Press, 1982.
2. Chengdu Medical School, ed. *Lecture Notes on the Theory of Feverish Diseases* (Wen ping hsueh chiang i, 溫病學講義). Shanghai: Science and Technology Press, 1978.
3. Hsu, Hong-yen, *The Essentials of Conformation in Chinese Medicine* (Chung i pien cheng kang yao, 中醫辨證綱要). Taipei: New Drug Press, 1977.
4. Hsu, Hong-yen and Hsu, Chau-shin, *Commonly Used Chinese Herb Formulas with Illustrations.* Los Angeles: Oriental Healing Arts Institute, 1980.
5. Hsu, Hong-yen and Peacher, William G. tr. *Chen's History of Chinese Medicine.* Los Angeles: Oriental Healing Arts Institute, 1980.
6. Nanching Medical School, ed. *Exposition of Feverish Diseases* (Wen ping hsueh shih i, 溫病學釋義). Shanghai: People's Health Press, 1982.
7. Ou-Yang, Chi *Lecture on Chinese Medical Classics* (Chung i ching dian chiang ko, 中醫經典講課). Hunan: Science and Technology Press, 1982.
8. Traditional Chinese Medical Research Institute and Kuang-tung Institute of Traditional Chinese Medicine, eds. *Dictionary of Traditional Chinese Medical Terms*

(Chung i ming tsu su yu tsu tien, 中醫名詞術語詞典). Hong Kong: Business Affair Press, 1975.

9. Wang, Chi-ju *Views on Feverish Diseases* (Wen pien chu yen, 溫病芻言). Tien-chin: Science and Technology Press, 1981.

10. Wu, Chu-tung *Detailed Analysis of Feverish Diseases* (Wen ping tiao pien, 溫病條辨). Taipei: Whirlwind Press, 1967.

Appendix

Formulas Not Listed in *Commonly Used Chinese Herb Formulas with Illustrations**

Unit: gram

Agastache and Polyporus Combination
Huo-pu-hsia-ling-tang (藿朴夏苓湯)
(*Detailed Analysis of Feverish Diseases,* 溫病條辨)

Agastache 6.0	Pinellia 5.0	Magnolia bark 3.0
Hoelen 10.0	Apricot seed 10.0	Coix 12.0
Cluster 2.0	Polyporus 5.0	Prepared soybean 10.0
Alisma 5.0		

Allium and Platycodon Combination
Tsung-shih-chieh-keng-tang (葱豉桔梗湯)
(*On Common Febrile Diseases,* 通俗傷寒論)

Allium 3.0	Soybean 9.0	Gardenia 6.0
Platycodon 3.0	Mentha 3.0	Bamboo leaf 9.0
Forsythia 4.5	Licorice 1.8	

Antelope Horn Powder
Ling-yang-chiao-fen (羚羊角粉)
(*Prescriptions for Saving Lives,* 濟生方)

Antelope horn 1.5	*Tuhuo* 1.5	Jujube 1.5
Acanthopanax 1.5	Coix 1.5	Siler 1.5
Tang-kuei 1.5	Cnidium 1.5	*Fushen* 1.5
Apricot seed 1.5	Saussurea 1.5	Licorice 0.6

*If the listed formulas are not available, similar prescriptions can be substituted.

Antelope Horn and Gambir Combination
Ling-yang-kou-teng-tang (羚羊鈎藤湯)
(*On Common Febrile Diseases,* 通俗傷寒論)

Antelope horn powder 1.0	Morus leaf 6.0	Fritillaria 12.0
Chrysanthemum 10.0	Rehmannia 15.0	Gambir 10.0
	Peony 10.0	Licorice 2.0
	Bamboo 15.0	*Fushen* 10.0

Apricot, Coix, and Cluster Combination
San-jen-tang (三仁湯)
(*Detailed Analysis of Feverish Diseases,* 溫病條辨)

Apricot seed 10.0	Talc 20.0	Tetrapanax 6.0
Bamboo leaf 6.0	Magnolia bark 6.0	Coix 20.0
Pinellia 10.0	Cluster 3.0	

Areca Seed and Magnolia Combination
Ta-yuan-yin (達原飲)
(*Exposition on Feverish Diseases,* 溫疫論)

Areca seed 6.0	Magnolia bark 3.0	*Tsao-kuo* 3.0
Anemarrhena 6.0	Peony 3.0	Scute 4.5
Licorice 3.0		

Astragalus and Wheat Combination**
Huang-chi-ku-piao-tang (黃耆固表湯)

Astragalus 30.0	Wheat 30.0	Mahuang root 10.0
Licorice 5.0	White atractylodes 9.0	Schizandra 6.0

Chih-shih and Rhubarb Combination
Chih-shih-tao-chih-tang (枳實導滯湯)
(*On Common Febrile Diseases,* 通俗傷寒論)

Hawthorn 9.0	Red yeast ferment 9.0	*Chih-shih* 6.0
Rhubarb 4.5		Areca seed 4.5
Forsythia 4.5	Akebia 2.4	Szechuan coptis 1.8
Magnolia bark 4.5	Lithospermum 9.0	Licorice 1.5

**Formula originated by author.

Ching-hao and Scute Combination
Hao-chin-ching-tan-tang (蒿芩淸膽湯)
(*On Common Febrile Diseases,* 通俗傷寒論)

Ching-hao 6.0	Bamboo 9.0	Pinellia 4.5
Hoelen 9.0	Scute 4.5	*Chih-ko* 4.5
Citrus 4.5	Talc and Indigo Formula 9.0	

Ching-hao and Turtle Shell Combination**
Ching-hao-pieh-chia-chien (青蒿別甲煎)

Ching-hao 6.0	Turtle shell 6.0	Lycium bark 12.0
Anemarrhena 10.0	Trichosanthes root 12.0	

Coptis and Acorus Combination
Wangs-lien-pu-yin (王氏連朴飲)
(*The Longitude and Latitude of Feverish Diseases,* 溫熱經緯)

Coptis 3.0	Magnolia bark 6.0	Gardenia 9.0
Pinellia 3.0	Soybean 9.0	Acorus 3.0

Coptis and Elsholtzia Combination
Huang-lien-hsiang-ju-yin (黃連香薷飲)
(*Collection of Prescriptions with Exposition,* 醫方集解)

Elsholtzia 6.0	Magnolia bark 3.0	Hyacinth bean 3.0
Coptis 1.5		

Forsythia and Mentha Combination
Chiao-ho-tang (翹荷湯)
(*Detailed Analysis of Feverish Diseases,* 溫病條辨)

Forsythia 4.5	Mentha 4.5	Licorice 3.0
Platycodon 6.0	Gardenia bark 4.5	Mung bean husk 6.0

Gelatin and Yolk Combination
Ah-chiao-chi-tzu-huang-tang (阿膠雞子黃湯)
(*On Common Febrile Diseases,* 通俗傷寒論)

Gelatin 6.0	White peony 10.0	Haliotis 15.0
Gambir 6.0	Rehmannia 12.0	Licorice 2.0
Oyster shell 12.0	Star jasmine 10.0	Yolk of two eggs
Fushen 12.0		

Ginseng, Schizandra, and Ophiopogon Formula
Sheng-mai-san (生脈散)
(*On Differentiation of Internal and External Injuries,* 內外傷辨惑論)

Ginseng 12.0	Schizandra 6.0	Ophiopogon 12.0

Glehnia and Ophiopogon Combination
I-wei-tang (益胃湯)
(*Detailed Analysis of Feverish Diseases,* 溫病條辨)

Glehnia 12.0	Ophiopogon 12.0	Rehmannia 12.0
Polygonatum 10.0	Crystal sugar 20.0	

Glehnia and Rehmannia Combination
I-kuang-chien (一貫煎)
(*Medical Lectures of Liou Chou,* 柳州醫話)

Glehnia 10.0	Rehmannia 2.0	Ophiopogon 10.0
Lycium fruit 10.0	Melia 5.0	*Tang-kuei* 10.0

Gypsum and Anemarrhena Combination
Shih-chuan-ku-han-chiu-pu-tang (十全苦寒救補湯)
(*On Feverish and Fever Diseases,* 溫熱論)

Gypsum 24.0	Anemarrhena 18.0	Scute 18.0
Phellodendron 15.0	Rhinoceros horn 15.0	*Chih-shih* 15.0
Coptis 9.0	Mirabilitum 9.0	Rhubarb 9.0
Magnolia bark 3.0		

Gypsum and Anemone Combination **
Tou-je-chuan-chi-tang (透熱轉氣湯)

Gypsum 30.0	Anemarrhena 10.0	Silkworm 10.0
Cicada 5.0	Lonicera 30.0	Forsythia 30.0
Talc 12.0	Gardenia 10.0	Bamboo 12.0
Rhinoceros horn 0.6	Antelope horn 0.6	Tabasheer 10.0
Anemone 10.0	Bos and Curcuma Formula 1 pill	

Gypsum and Hoelen Combination
Chu-shu-tiao-yuan-fa (祛暑調元法)
(*On Seasonal Diseases,* 時病論)

Gypsum 12.0	Hoelen 9.0	Talc 9.0
Pinellia 3.0	Ginseng 6.0	Ophiopogon 6.0

Licorice 1.8 Platycodon small amount

Gypsum and Lycium Bark Combination**
Ching-je-ku-piao-tang (清熱固表湯)

Gypsum 30.0	Lycium bark 12.0	Wheat 30.0
Anemarrhena 10.0	Oryza 30.0	

Gypsum and Moutan Combination
Ching-wen-pai-tu-yin (清瘟敗毒飲)
(*An Experience of Epidemic Skin Eruptions*, 疫疹一得)

Gypsum 30.0-120.0	Moutan 10.0	Rehmannia 30.0
Coptis 10.0	Gardenia 10.0	Scute 10.0
Anemarrhena 10.0	Forsythia 15.0	Peony 10.0
Scrophularia 10.0	Licorice 3.0	Platycodon 5.0
Bamboo leaf 20 pieces		Rhinoceros 2.0-4.0

Gypsum and Oryza Combination
Hua-pan-tang (化斑湯)
(*Detailed Analysis of Feverish Diseases*, 溫病條辨)

Gypsum 30.0	Oryza 12.0	Anemarrhena 12.0
Licorice 4.5	Scrophularia 12.0	Rhinoceros 0.6

Gypsum and Rhubarb Combination
Hsuan-pai-cheng-chi-tang (宣白承氣湯)
(*Detailed Analysis of Feverish Diseases*, 溫病條辨)

Gypsum 15.0	Rhubarb 9.0	Apricot seed powder 6.0
Trichosanthes bark 4.5		

Gypsum, Rhubarb, and Anemarrhena Combination**
Pai-hu-cheng-chi-tang (白虎承氣湯)

Gypsum	Anemarrhena	Rhubarb
Chih-shih	Magnolia bark	Lonicera
Forsythia	Mirabilitum	

Haliotis and Gentiana Combination**
Tung-chiao-hsi-feng-tang (通竅熄風湯)

Haliotis 30.0	Gentiana 10.0	Gambir 12.0
Scorpion 5.0	Gypsum 30.0	Silkworm 10.0

Tabasheer 10.0	Anemone 10.0	Curcuma 10.0
Lonicera 30.0	Forsythia 15.0	Anemarrhena 10.0
Phellodendron 10.0	Antelope horn 0.6	Rhinoceros horn 0.6
Bos and Curcuma Formula 1 pill		

Hoelen Four Herb Formula
Szu-ling-san (四苓散)
(*Exposition on Feverish Plagues,* 溫疫論)

Hoelen 4.0	Alisma 4.0	Polyporus 4.0
White atractylodes 4.0		

Lonicera and Anemarrhena Combination**
Ching-shu-chieh-tu-tang (清暑解毒湯)

Gypsum 30.0	Reed 30.0	Silkworm 10.0
Cicada 5.0	Mentha 5.0	Lonicera 20.0
Forsythia 20.0	Talc 18.0	Licorice 3.0
Anemarrhena 10.0	Lotus leaf 12.0	Watermelon skin 30.0

Lonicera and Gypsum Combination**
Liang-hsueh-pai-tu-tang (涼血敗毒湯)

Gypsum 30.0	Anemarrhena 10.0	Moutan 10.0
Lonicera 30.0	Carthamus 30.0	Forsythia 30.0
Coptis 6.0	Scute 10.0	Rehmannia 30.0
Talc 12.0	Gardenia 10.0	Scrophularia 15.0
Woolly grass 30.0	Rhinoceros horn 0.6	Antelope horn 0.6

Lonicera and Lotus Leaf Combination
Ching-lo-yin (清絡飲)
(*Detailed Analysis of Feverish Diseases,* 溫病條辨)

Lonicera 6.0	Lotus leaf 6.0	Watermelon skin 6.0
Luffa peel 6.0	Bamboo leaf 6.0	Hyacinth flower with stem 1 pill

Lonicera Stem and Clematis Combination**
Su-lo-chu-feng-tang (舒絡祛風湯)

Morus leaf 10.0	Morus branch 20.0	Gentiana 6.0
Bamboo 12.0	Lonicera 15.0	Silkworm 10.0

Clematis 5.0

Magnolia and Agastache Combination
Fang-hsiang-hua-cho-fa (芳香化濁法)
(*On Seasonal Diseases,* 時病論)

Magnolia bark 2.4	Agastache 3.0	Pinellia 4.5
Citrus 4.5	Lotus leaf 9.0	Areca husk 3.0
Eupatorium 3.0		

Morus and Bupleurum Combination**
Sang-chai-yin (桑柴飲)

Morus 10.0	Bupleurum 5.0	Mentha 5.0
Scute 10.0	Pinellia 10.0	Lonicera 12.0
Forsythia 12.0		

Morus and Linum Formula
Sang-ma-wan (桑麻丸)
(*Collection of Prescriptions with Exposition,* 醫方集解)

Morus 40.0	Linum 10.0	Honey 4.0

(Linum can be substituted by an equal amount of cannabis seed)

Pear Five Juice Combination
Wu-chih-yin (五汁飲)
(*Detailed Analysis of Feverish Diseases,* 溫病條辨)

Pear juice	Reed juice	Ophiopogon juice
Lotus juice	Water chestnut juice	

Peony and Coptis Combination
Tao-chih-cheng-chi-tang (導赤承氣湯)
(*Detailed Analysis of Feverish Diseases,* 溫病條辨)

Peony 9.0	Rhubarb 9.0	Coptis 6.0
Phellodendron 6.0	Rehmannia 15.0	Mirabilitum 3.0

Peony and Gelatin Formula
Ta-ting-feng-chu (大定風珠)
(*Detailed Analysis of Feverish Diseases,* 溫病條辨)

Peony 18.0	Gelatin 9.0	Licorice 12.0
Rehmannia 18.0	Ophiopogon 18.0	Oyster shell 12.0
Hemp 6.0	Tortoise shell 12.0	Turtle shell 12.0

Schizandra 6.0	Yolk of two eggs	

Persica and Biota Formula
Wu-jen-wan (五仁丸)
(*Effective Formulas Tested by Physicians for Generations,* 世醫得效方)

Persica seed 9.0	Biota seed 9.0	Pine seed 3.0
Apricot seed 12.0	Citrus 6.0	Japanese plum 6.0

Phellodendron, Anemarrhena, and Cinnamon Formula
Tzu-shen-wan (滋腎丸)
(*Secret Recipe of the Orchid Room,* 蘭室秘藏)

Phellodendron 10.0	Anemarrhena 10.0	Cinnamon 1.0

Pleione and Nutgalls Formula
Yu-shu-tan (玉樞丹)
(*A Medical Book Worth Pieces of Jade,* 生玉心書)

Pleione 60.0	Nutgalls 30.0	Knoxia 45.0
Lathyrol spurge 30.0	Realgar 6.0	Musk 9.0
Cinnabar 12.0		

Polygonatum and Mahuang Combination
Wei-jui-tang (葳蕤湯)
(*Prescriptions Worth A Thousand,* 千金方)

Polygonatum 6.0	Mahuang 6.0	*Tuhuo* 6.0
Cynanchum 6.0	Apricot seed 6.0	Cnidium 6.0
Licorice 6.0	Birthwort 6.0	Gypsum 9.0

Rehmannia and Lophatherum Combination
Tao-chih-ching-hsin-tang (導赤清心湯)
(*On Common Febrile Disease,* 通俗傷寒論)

Rehmannia 18.0	Lophatherum 4.5	*Fushen* 6.0
Moutan 6.0	Ophiopogon 4.5	Akebia 1.5
Talc and Cinnabar Formula 9.0	Lotus embryonic shoot 30 pieces	Bog rush 20 pieces

Rehmannia, Ophiopogon, and Scrophularia Combination
Tseng-yeh-tang (增液湯)

(*Detailed Analysis of Feverish Diseases,* 溫病條辨)

Rehmannia 30.0	Ophiopogon 30.0	Scrophularia 30.0

Rhinoceros Horn Powder
Hsi-chiao-fen (犀角粉)
(*Standards of Diagnosis and Treatment,* 證治準繩)

Rhinoceros 3.0	*Chih-ko* 3.0	Siler 2.0
Aquilaria 3.0	Perilla 4.0	Areca seed 4.0
Ophiopogon 4.0	Saussurea 2.0	Hoelen 4.0
Gypsum 8.0	Lophatherum 1 teaspoon	

Rhinoceros and Cinnabar Formula**
Huei-su-san (回蘇散)

Rhinoceros horn 1.0	Antelope horn 1.0	Musk 0.3
Bos 0.3	Borneol 0.3	Ambergris 0.3
Mentha 0.15	Pearl 0.3	Cinnabar 3.0
Succinum 3.0		

Rhinoceros and Lonicera Formula
Shen-hsi-tan (神犀丹)
(*The Longitude and Latitude of Feverish Diseases,* 溫熱經緯)

Rhinoceros horn 6.0	Acorus 6.0	Scute 6.0
Rehmannia 16.0	Lonicera 16.0	Forsythia 10.0
Isatis 9.0	Soybean 8.0	Scrophularia 7.0
Arnebia 4.0	Trichosanthes root 4.0	

Rhinoceros and Moutan Combination
Hsi-ti-ching-lo-yin (犀地清絡飲)
(*On Common Febrile Diseases,* 通俗傷寒論)

Rhinoceros horn 1.0	Moutan 6.0	Forsythia 4.5
Peony 4.5	Rehmannia 24.0	Persica 9 kernels

Some ginger and bamboo sap

Rhinoceros and Scrophularia Combination
Ching-ying-tang (清營湯)
(*Detailed Analysis of Feverish Diseases,* 溫病條辨)

Rehmannia 15.0	Scrophularia 10.0	Ophiopogon 10.0
Lonicera 10.0	Forsythia 10.0	Coptis 5.0

Salvia 6.0 | Bamboo leaf 3.0 | Rhinoceros horn 1.0

Schizonepeta, Siler, and Chiang-huo Combination**
Ching-fang-chieh-tu-yin (荆防解毒飲)
Schizonepeta 5.0 | Siler 5.0 | *Chiang-huo* 5.0
Lonicera 15.0 | Forsythia 15.0 | Perilla 5.0
Pinellia 10.0 | Citrus 5.0

Siler and Mentha Formula
Shuang-chieh-san (雙解散)
(*Prescriptions of Liu Ho-chien*, 劉河間方)
Siler 2.0 | Mentha 2.0 | Schizonepeta 2.0
Mahuang 2.0 | *Tang-kuei* 2.0 | Cnidium 2.0
Peony 2.0 | White atractylodes 2.0 | Forsythia 2.0
Gardenia 2.0 | Platycodon 3.0 | Rhubarb 2.0
Mirabilitum 2.0 | Talc 10.0 | Scute 3.0
Gypsum 12.0 | | Licorice 6.0

Silkworm and Rhubarb Formula
Sheng-chiang-san (升降散)
(*Detailed Analysis of Cold-Feverish Diseases*, 寒溫條辨)
Silkworm 6.0 | Cicada 3.0 | Rhubarb 12.0
Turmeric 1.0

Talc and Cinnabar Formula
I-yuan-san (益元散)
(*The Golden Mirror of Medicine*, 醫宗金鑑)
Talc 18.0 | Cinnabar 6.0 | Licorice 3.0

Talc and Licorice Formula
Liu-i-san (六一散)
(*Prescriptions of Liu Ho-chien*, 劉河間方)
Talc 18.0 | Licorice 3.0

Talc and Scute Formula
Kan-lu-hsiao-tu-tan (甘露消毒丹)
(*The Longitude and Latitude of Feverish Diseases*, 溫熱經緯)
Talc 30.0 | Scute 9.0 | Capillaris 18.0

Akebia 6.0
Acorus 6.0
Fritillaria 6.0
Forsythia 10.0
Mentha 5.0
Cluster 3.0
Agastache 3.0
Belamcanda 5.0

Talc, Calcite, and Gypsum Combination
San-shih-tang (三石湯)
(*Detailed Analysis of Feverish Diseases,* 溫熱條辨)
Talc 9.0
Calcite 9.0
Gypsum 15.0
Apricot seed 9.0
Bamboo 6.0
Lonicera 9.0
Tetrapanax 9.0

Formula Index

Formula Index
Chinese

Index

The Theory of Feverish Diseases and Its Clinical Applications

- *Enumeration of feverish diseases and their etiologies*
- *Diagnosis and treatment of feverish diseases*
- *Examination of the relationships between feverish diseases*

Other Publications of the Oriental Healing Arts Institute

CHINESE HERBAL MEDICINE AND THE PROBLEMS OF AGING

In his book Dr. Terashi, a Western-trained physician who went on to study traditional Chinese medicine, discusses the diagnoses and herbal therapy for a number of debilitating and disabling diseases. Once associated almost exclusively with older persons, many of these maladies now occur with more frequency in younger people. Dr. Terashi's excellent case histories present a comprehensive view of such chronic and recalcitrant diseases as heart and circulatory diseases, respiratory disorders, liver and kidney disease, metabolic and skin disorders, gynecological problems, and sexual dysfunction. Anyone wanting to learn more about effective medical treatments devoid of danger or harmful side effects will find this an invaluable book. *Terashi Bokuso, M.D. 1984. 238 Pages. Paper $12.00.*

THIRTY YEARS OF KANPO

Dr. Otsuka's unique approach is his use of case studies to share his more than thirty years of accumulated knowledge of medicine, both Western and Oriental. Health care professionals will find the subsequent blend of medical theory fascinating as well as extremely valuable. The deeply personal nature of the discussions actually makes the book an autobiography of a practicing physician. The cases reveal the integrity, competence, and compassion of a good man as he goes about his business healing and giving aid to the sick. *Otsuka Keisetsu, M.D. 1984. 442 Pages. Paper $18.00.*

COMMONLY USED CHINESE HERB FORMULAS WITH ILLUSTRATIONS

This book contains an extensive compilation of the herbal formulas commonly prescribed by physicians who follow the Chinese herbal tradition. Twenty-four categories of formulas are presented according to their pharmaceutical action: emetics, purgatives, anthelmintics, *ch'i* formulas, sedatives, etc. Included in each formula's entry are its ingredients, indications, and discriminatory symptoms, plus an anatomical diagram showing the targets of treatment. *Hsu, Hong-yen, Ph.D., & Hsu, Chau-shin, Ph.D., 1982. 671 Pages. Hardback $25.00. Paper $19.95.*